Ruth Field is no professional fitness guru. She is, however, a keen runner who, while pregnant with twins and under doctor's orders not to run, decided to write this book as an outlet for her frustration. She never dreamed anyone would actually read it. Let alone buy it.

Praise for *Run Fat B!tch Run*

'If you're stuck in an exercise rut, this book will give you a rather rude kick up the backside . . . it certainly shamed us into lacing up our Nikes!'

Closer

'Amusingly vicious . . . Excellent advice all round'

Emma Thompson

'Ruth is an inspiring running-buddy . . . By the time I unpack my summer wardrobe, I'm sure my inner Grit Doctor will be my best friend'

Daily Express

'A witty, no-nonsense read, it had us dusting off our trainers within seconds. Trust us when we say you'll be up and running in no time at all'

Grazia

By Ruth Field

Run Fat B!tch Run
Get Your Sh!t Together

RUN FAT B!TCH RUN

BY RUTH FIELD

AND INTRODUCING
THE GRIT DOCTOR

sphere

SPHERE

First published in Great Britain in 2012 by Sphere
This paperback edition published in 2014 by Sphere

A CIP catalogue record for this book
is available from the British Library.

ISBN 978-0-7515-5398-7

Typeset in Bembo by M Rules
Printed and bound in Great Britain by
Clays Ltd, St Ives plc

Papers used by Sphere are from well-managed forests
and other responsible sources.

MIX
Paper from
responsible sources
FSC® C104740

Sphere
An imprint of
Little, Brown Book Group
100 Victoria Embankment
London EC4Y 0DY

An Hachette UK Company
www.hachette.co.uk

www.littlebrown.co.uk

For Olly, and for my grandfather, Cyril Field.

CONTENTS

PART 3 NOW WHAT?

PART 4 THE MARATHON PLAN

WHO IS THE GRIT DOCTOR?

I am The Grit Doctor. I am a ruthless no-nonsense motivator who will force you to do the things you don't want to do. I will bully you into submission and then inspire you to heights greater than you thought possible. I am the voice you will tune into when you are feeling at your most lazy and ineffectual and the one who will help you ignore the deafening call of the sofa. I am the voice you need to listen to and obey.

Once you learn to understand and enjoy the voice of The Grit Doctor, it won't be long before you can tune into it whenever you choose and use it to push yourself forward when you might otherwise give up. The voice of The Grit Doctor is what you've been missing in your life. You just didn't know it until now.

A GRIT DOCTOR HEALTH WARNING:

The exercise programmes in this book are intended for those in reasonable physical and mental health – if you have a genuine medical condition, an underlying injury, are pregnant or have any other health concerns, for the love of God consult your GP before starting out. However, under no circumstances invent health concerns or problems and use them as an excuse to skive running sessions.

YOUR POINTLESS PLEDGE

I _____ do solemnly declare and accept that I am a FAT BITCH and I want to do something about it. I promise not to waste any more valuable fat-busting time in buying fancy equipment, joining expensive gyms and exercise classes or filling in charts with weights and measurements. I will no longer be seduced by faddy diets. I will stop making excuses for myself and, holding hands with my inner bitch, I will haul my fat arse off the sofa and get out of the front door.

I swear on my mother's life to do as The Grit Doctor tells me and at all times to retain my sense of humour.

Signed:

Dated:

PART 1

RUNNING

INTRODUCTION

This book is not for the committed fitness freak. Nor is it meant for the super-motivated. I am not here to help you to acheive a perfect 'beach body' or sculpt your deltoids. If you already have the body you want, and that includes those of you who are fat and blissfully happy just as much as the super-slim and toned among you, congratulations. You don't need to read any further.

This book is specifically designed for those of you who are *unhappy with your body*. Those of you who feel stuck and unable to commit to anything by way of exercise or diet for long enough to see any results. It is designed to shake you out of your torpor, get you up off the sofa and embracing a new way of being.

The good news is that nothing in this book is rocket science. In fact, a great deal of it is common sense. *So why do I need to read it, then?* I hear you ask. Well, knowing something is common sense is all well and good, but when it is buried under layers of self-delusion, it's not always that easy to act on. You know that eating healthily is common sense too, don't you? And yet that cream cake makes you dribble with desire and you happily bypass the fruit bowl to get at it. So don't be fooled into thinking you know it all already. You don't.

When I say it's not rocket science, what I mean is that if you're looking for the latest high-tech, Gwyneth Paltrow-approved weight-loss programme, you've come to the wrong place. This book follows a basic formula: run, eat less rubbish, lose weight. Simple. But don't confuse simple with easy. Straightforward, yes. Easy, no.

Running is simple in the sense that it is entirely natural and instinctive. Just watch the way that any child, freed from the protective grasp of a parent's hand, joyfully runs about with complete and utter abandon. Nothing could be more natural. But while it is a simple activity, *easy* it isn't. Certainly not when you're doing it as a self-conscious adult as opposed to during a game of kiss-chase in the school playground. So in order to rediscover this natural gift that you were born with, you will need education, discipline and commitment. But don't panic, The Grit Doctor will be with you all the way and will help you dig deep and find all three.

Before we get under way, there are three concepts you must take on board. Immediately.

1. **You need to be taught how to run**. It is not quite as simple as merely going outside and giving it a whirl.

2. When it comes to food and weight-loss, the bottom line is this: **your run will be your diet**. Quite literally.

3. This final point is critical: in order to hear my message clearly, **you will need to make friends with your inner bitch**. My own inner bitch is The Grit Doctor and I'm lending her to you for the duration of this book. I hope you will come to know and love her, and ultimately adopt her, adapt her and make her your own.

Now I know that this whole Grit Doctor thing is in danger of making me sound like some kind of nutter, but really I am just naming that voice we all have inside our heads. Yours may be lying dormant, or suffocating under your excess weight, but *it is there*. That nagging little voice which makes you feel just a tad uncomfortable about helping yourself to another biscuit or ignoring the wet laundry in order to watch one more episode of *Glee*. You know, the one you usually ignore. Well, not any more. One of the things I am going to try and help you do is to listen much more carefully to that voice – amplify it in fact – until it really gets in your face.

The Grit Doctor will be with you throughout this book. She'll be there, holding up a mirror when you slump back onto the sofa, sighing that this all sounds too much like hard work as you reach for the Dairy Milk. She will motivate, inspire, and yes, even bully you into making the necessary changes in your life. Sometimes you will hate her. One day you'll want to shout back and show her who's boss. And when that happens, you'll know you've turned a corner and found your own inner bitch.

If tapping into this pool of negativity seems odd, or even unhealthy, let me say this by way of reassurance. The Grit Doctor is a *device* I have harnessed to help motivate myself to do the things I'd often really rather not. She is there only when I need her. I can say with absolute certainty that if I employed Grit Doctor tactics in all areas of my life *all of the time*, I would be extremely unpopular and probably divorced. But here's the thing: I know that with The Grit Doctor's help I can power through the boring bits of life with relative ease.

So I'm sure you've figured out by now that The Grit Doctor is not going to dress this up as 'fun' and make you feel good about yourself if there's plainly nothing to feel good about. I don't want to waste my energy or yours filling your head with nonsense about how much fun running is and how great you look. The former is a lie and the fact that you are reading this book ought to give you a clue about the latter. I want you to be honest with yourself, hard on yourself even. Because there is no magic pill and none of it is easy. *Stop wanting things to be easy*. Once you accept – and I mean *really* accept – that life is not easy, it actually becomes a lot more manageable because you stop resisting the hard work, and find the determination

and grit that is required in order to achieve anything worth-
while. This is going to be hard. *But* – and this is the crucial
BUT – **you are going to start *enjoying* hard. Embracing
hard. Hard is going to be the new black.**

Once you have 'got it' and achieved your desired weight,
you will only need to find three forty-minute free periods
each week in order to look great and eat well *for the rest of
your life.* And you will have it forever and *wherever* you find
yourself: on holiday, in the countryside, in the city, at your
mum's or on your way back from work, because it only
involves putting on your shoes and stepping outside for forty
minutes. No fancy equipment, no having to get yourself
somewhere else first, negotiating your way through rush-
hour traffic or the ball-ache of public transport. You are
always only two minutes away from getting the job done,
which is putting on your trainers and getting out of the front
door.

FAST TRACK OR SLOW COACH?

Some of you will find this easier than others. Perhaps the
seed of motivation to get fit or lose weight has already
been sown and is just waiting for a Big Bang to bring it to
life. So if you're already feeling inspired, just jump forward to
page 59 where you'll find a simple step-by-step guide to getting started – far be it from me to hold you back if you're

already raring to go. And you can always come back and read the other bits later.

But for those of you who quite literally need dragging out from under the duvet, the Slow Coach approach is tailor-made for you. Don't be embarrassed – the fact that you've bought this book is a step in the right direction and you'll be up and running in no time at all. You'll probably need to read everything straight through, including the more detailed beginners' programme, designed specifically for chronic couch potatoes. The Grit Doctor is not shy of hand-holding and will walk you through all the necessary steps. You may start off as a Slow Coach and discover midway through that you want to Fast Track or vice versa. This is also fine.

OK bitches, let's get moving.

Ruth

I started running when I was twenty-four. I'd given up all exercise at university, having previously been really into sport, and I knew that something was missing from my life. I was also single again after a long relationship, so maybe that had something to do with it too.

I had begun training as a barrister and my pupil master insisted on eating a proper lunch on a daily basis, by which I mean a curry, a Chinese or something equally naughty and spectacularly calorific. Bless him, it was the only meal of the day that he 'took', as he would say. Unfortunately it meant my appetite soon spiralled out of control as I continued to eat a huge evening meal and a hearty breakfast, without doing any exercise at all except dashing to and from court. I immediately started to pile on the pounds. (Someone recently pointed out to me that I have never been fat and I think it is only fair to own up to this. I have never been overweight in the strictest sense of the word. But, like most women, there have been times in my life when I have definitely needed to lose a few pounds and this was one of them. I was three-quarters of a stone over my usual weight, my clothes were getting really tight and when I looked in the mirror I saw the makings of a very FAT BITCH indeed.)

It was around this time that a great friend of mine, Jane – who was not known for her sporting prowess – announced in the pub that she was going to run the London Marathon. I was stunned, as were all our mates. Jane was comfortably the least likely of all of us to do something like this, which of course made her announcement all the more impressive. I was beside myself with envy and immediately said I would run with her (mainly to impress the audience), having no idea how to run or what a marathon was all about.

I had six months to figure it out. What kept me going in those early days was the knowledge that I couldn't back out after making such a public proclamation and signing up to run for a charity. I was fully committed to running the bloody marathon and quitting was not an option. And I knew I didn't have a hope in hell if I didn't start training.

I can honestly say I hated every single one of those early runs. I was shocked at how hard it was and ashamed at how unfit I had become, as I struggled to run for even five minutes without feeling like I was on the verge of a heart attack. It was incredibly difficult and not helped by the dreadful route I chose – laps of Clapham Common, a flat and featureless landscape which left me feeling totally uninspired. It didn't occur to me to get a book on running or to ask for help. I just kept at it, with The Grit Doctor always breathing down my neck, telling me that if I didn't sort myself out I'd be a total loser and that Jane would beat me. Which she did, by the way. (Ten years on and it still pains me to acknowledge that.)

So that's how it started. I had needed to do something to burn off those lunches and then my competitive spirit was awakened one day in the pub. I had no idea at the time what a great, life-long gift Jane and my pupil master had indirectly given me. I had no intention of becoming a runner, I just wanted to lose some weight, run this race and then get back to my normal life again. What I didn't know then was how running would ultimately transform so many other areas of my life. No longer would I need to complain about the cost of a gym membership or find time to join a club. I would have something to do all by myself for the rest of my life. Something that would satisfy me completely.

There was never one moment for me when it all 'clicked'. There was just before and after I ran. I really only became a runner after that first marathon, because beforehand I really hated it: the training, the stress, the knowledge that

I wasn't nearly fit enough and the constant nagging feeling I might not do myself justice. I certainly wasn't planning on running after it and I didn't run for a couple of weeks once it was over … I couldn't anyway, my toes were in tatters. But to my surprise, I found myself really missing how it had made me feel. I dug out my trainers and hit the park and that was the moment that really marked the beginning of my life as a runner – it felt like I was choosing to get out there in a way I hadn't before. So having thought I wouldn't want to run ever again, I soon found I couldn't live without it.

THE GRIT DOCTOR SAYS:

YOU MAY NEVER ACTUALLY ENJOY RUNNING. If you are one of the lucky ones you will reach a stage during *some* runs when everything feels so right that you almost forget you are running. You are running 'in the zone' and that is a real pleasure. But it doesn't always happen and it doesn't always last. You will hate some runs from start to finish. What you ENJOY is less the run itself and more what the practice of running is enabling you to do in the rest of your life. The pleasure you really get from running is FROM THE FACT THAT YOU HAVE RUN; that you put your trainers

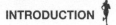

on, braved the great outdoors and actually did it, in spite of all the excuses you could think of not to.

Running requires an effort every time. It is very important to understand and accept this at the start to avoid unnecessary disappointment and motivation meltdown.

1

GETTING SHIT DONE

Running makes you rich . . .

Well, not exactly. What I mean is that it is a very cheap
hobby. In fact, it is essentially totally free, requiring little
financial investment on your part. Bar the cost of the
occasional new pair of trainers, it does not involve buying
fancy new clothes, new equipment or expensive
membership fees. You can even run without shoes if you
have to; indeed, running barefoot on a beautiful beach at
sunrise is to be recommended at least once in your life.
Plus, because it makes you so much more effective at
work, you probably will end up making more money!

AN ASSIGNMENT FROM THE GRIT DOCTOR:
THE 'WHEN I'M THIN' LIST

Make a list of all the things you have promised
to do when you are thin.

For example:

When I am thin I will . . .

- Buy – and wear – a body-con dress
- Apply for my dream job
- Sign up for a charity 5km and actually *run* it
- Ask out the hot guy in Starbucks
- Go on a beach holiday without having to
  wear a kaftan
- Marry George Clooney

The Grit Doctor is not a fan of lists – they are,
quite frankly, faffing in disguise, and wasted time
that would be better spent actually doing or acting
on the stuff on the list. (No, you don't need to
write another list in order to work out what it is
that you need to do. Put down your pen. Now.)
Give up 'to do' lists. Take up 'getting shit done'.
But I digress. The point of this exercise is extremely
important. NOW THAT YOU HAVE WRITTEN YOUR
LIST, RIP IT UP AND THROW IT AWAY. MAKE IT
THE LAST LIST THAT YOU EVER WRITE

'When I am thin I will ...' is one of the biggest and most dangerous delusions out there. It is, in fact, keeping you fat. Thin doesn't just happen and it certainly doesn't just happen if you have been overweight for a long time. It is extremely difficult, not to mention monstrously dull, committing to diet after diet after diet in an attempt to lose weight.

Just ask yourself how many times you have started a diet before? Be honest. How many Mondays started out with the best of intentions? Drinking gallons of water, eating rice cakes and apples, feeling vaguely faint by going-home time, getting to about Wednesday and then caving in and eating a slice of cake? OK, maybe you managed a few weeks before the cake eating began, but eventually those weeks of good behaviour were completely wasted. Or, maybe you lost a stone on a great diet but over the rest of the year it crept back on and when you weighed yourself after Crimbo, what do you know? Back to square one. *I know it is hard*. Losing weight is really, really hard, especially if you are going about it in the 'dieting' way.

The thing is, you have almost certainly set yourself impossibly high standards when it comes to the size and weight you need to be before you can do and have all the things on your 'when I am thin' list. The idea that only when you are thin you will be able to do x, y and z – including exercising – is actually a major factor in keeping the weight on. The fear that you *can't* do something because you are overweight is paralysing.

The only way to lose weight effectively and forever is through a committed exercise routine and, through that, *changing your attitude to food*. **Exercise is the real key to weight-loss, not food**. The whole concept of a 'diet' is that it has an end point: 'Lose X pounds in X number of weeks!' It is all a complete con. It is almost impossible to lose weight permanently through 'dieting' because when the diet ends you go back to what you ate before and the weight creeps back on. Crash diets are even worse. Losing an enormous amount of weight in a short space of time for a special occasion puts your body and mind under great strain and you'll soon revert back to your old ways as soon as the wedding dress/bikini/killer date-night dress comes off.

Starting a diet – even a good one – is a very difficult way to solve any weight issue because it addresses only one factor inside an enormously intricate problem. Don't get me wrong, what you are eating is undoubtedly part of the issue but it is *only a part of it*. I'm no psychologist, but it's well-known that eating is a very emotional thing. Your reasons for eating, your state of mind, your happiness levels, your body's learnt expectation of what you are going to put into it, your ideas about what it means to be hungry or thirsty, when and how you feel satisfied, and your bad habits all contribute to what you put in your mouth. Trying to turn yourself into a rice-cake-munching waif on a Monday morning, when up until Sunday night you have been used to takeaway pizza and Haribos is going to be impossible for your confused body. You will feel faint and weird and just plain starving hungry, and will inevitably fall off the wagon.

A MESSAGE FROM THE GRIT DOCTOR:
STOP FEELING DEPRESSED ABOUT BEING FAT AND START DOING SOMETHING ABOUT IT. GO OUTSIDE AND START WALKING.

Throw away the diet books. For the moment you can keep the contents of your fridge and cupboards and continue to eat in exactly the same way as you always have. Your current eating habits are not important – they are entirely secondary and *much less critical* than getting you outside and running. It is vital to your success not to do too many things at once. So your priority right now, your *only* priority, is running. Focus all your energy on this one thing; not the new clothes, new trainers, new body, new you, new anything. Forget buying anything new, just use what you have for the moment. Get yourself outdoors and start moving. That is all you need to do to start losing weight. Keep the rest of your life the same for now and simply concentrate on getting to grips with the basics of running. I know this is hard but it is not as hard as buying, preparing, cooking and eating a restricted diet three times a day and spending at least fifty per cent of the rest of the day fanta-sising about what you would rather be eating. I reckon that must take up a good few hours of your day at least. And it is all time wasted.

Learning to run, on the other hand, is an hour-and-a-half a day, tops – I know that sounds like a lot but it's an investment and I promise that you won't regret it. Plus, it's double-bubble – it acts as fitness time but *also* diet time, and there are a million other tangential benefits, too. For you Slow Coaches that means you get a whole lot more bang for your buck . . .

THE GRIT DOCTOR SAYS:

You may be feeling an urge to get started. If so, you must capitalise on this immediately and skip to the Six-Step Programme in chapter 3 and begin Step 1 without further ado. YOU DO NOT NEED TO DO ANYTHING ELSE FIRST. You can always read the preceding chapters on the loo or in the bath after you've completed Step 1. The Grit Doctor is keen that you take advantage of any motivation you have as it arises. Go on then, get cracking.

For the rest of you, read on . . .

RUNNING IS THE ANSWER

Forget all that Pilates, yoga, Zumba ... even gym sessions. Forget all of it. You will never have the body you want, nor the mental strength and stamina required to maintain it, until you take on board and 'practise' that **running is the answer**. It is the only answer. No exceptions. Ahh, I hear you object, what about so and so, and so and so, who have perfect physiques and are not runners? Well, I'm not talking to a professional gymnast or ballet dancer, am I? And trust me, they all know the value of what I am telling you. All other exercise, at the level at which you are doing it, is invariably *less* than running. By which I mean it is not enough. Not enough to change you and your body in the sort of permanent way I have in mind. And so for the purposes of this book, ladies, lolling around on a Pilates ball or cocking your leg up in the air in an aerobics class doesn't count. Give it all up and devote yourself entirely to the practice of running for now.

Once you have mastered the art of running, you can add in a spot of yoga or indeed any sport to your fitness regime, although I recommend that you make it *as well as* rather than *instead of* running. But give it all up for now until you have 'got' running and are fully committed to its practice. Of course, if you work out religiously at the gym five times a week, every week (and spend that time actually exercising and not faffing about with equipment and ogling other bodies), you will get fit. But I believe I am addressing the average man or woman who remains overweight and can't understand why, when they are attending an aerobics class twice a week or playing five-a-side football at the weekend. You are simply not doing anywhere near enough fat-busting, cardiovascular exercise to change anything about your body and your weight. Forget about classes and designer sportswear, and all the time-wasting that surrounds them. Do something much more effective, something much more strenuous, something that will really, *really* burn away the excess flab – in a way and at a rate that nothing you have tried thus far has been able to.

WHY RUN?

Now, why is it that running is the answer? Well, it is different from all other forms of exercise, at the level at which you are doing them, because *it is much harder*. Not harder as in more complicated, but harder as in more physically strenuous. And because it is that much harder, ultimately it is that much more rewarding, both in terms of the dramatic physical changes to your body and indeed to your life in general. You only have to ask any of your friends who run regularly, or look at the lean mean body of any long-distance runner to see why. It requires discipline and commitment above and beyond other forms of exercise. It all has to come from you. There is no help or encouragement to be gleaned from an instructor or classmate, no under-floor heating or delicate scent of incense, and no one but yourself to get you motivated or to blame if you fail. The first ten minutes or so of each run is hellish *every* time. You are entirely at the mercy of the elements, there are no breaks midway through, no variation in the movement, no half-time oranges and no team banter. It is the ultimate physical challenge because, at first blush, it looks boring, repetitive, difficult, relentless, punishing and joyless. **Sounds fun? Ha. I told you it was hard, but remember, hard is going to be the NEW BLACK.**

But surely there's an easier way?

There isn't. The Grit Doctor would like to remind you, *again*, that embracing the fact that this is going to be hard is the only cure for the terminally unmotivated. The Grit Doctor suspects that you have become an expert at avoiding the hard things in life. You find yourself stuck in an exercise/weight rut from which you seem unable to escape and cannot understand why your lame efforts fail to yield spectacular results. You have come to expect that somehow you will get thin or fit 'the easy way' and keep starting a Pilates class or making it to the swimming pool once a month. You think that this is sufficient effort on your part. It isn't.

But look on the bright side, once you choose to follow The Grit Doctor and surrender to the idea that it will be hard, the world becomes your oyster. Hard is no longer something that you studiously avoid, but instead becomes something you know is necessary to get the results that you so desperately want. All the clichés back me up:

The *harder* the challenge, the greater the glory.
The *harder* the life, the sweeter the song.
The *harder* the conflict, the more glorious the triumph.

The good news is that once you have become a runner (and that does not mean once you have been on your first run – you *become a runner* when you have been at it for some time, when you are several months into running regularly) it won't be long before you no longer find it hard. Ultimately, you will need to create new levels of hard in order to challenge and stretch yourself further and you will come to enjoy this process. For now, just accept that running is hard and you are probably not going to enjoy it. But believe that there must be something in it – something pretty special – otherwise why are the parks and streets filled with runners at all times of the day and night as they keep coming back for more?

THE GRIT DOCTOR SAYS:

Spectacular results are only achieved through spectacular effort. No exceptions.

Perhaps a few of you have been totally put off by some of the points raised above. And maybe you have been running a couple of times and decided it *is* actually unbelievably boring, you got nothing out of it and vowed never to do it again. Be honest though, have you dismissed other forms of exercise after trying them out just the once, or given up on a diet after just two days? Have you *ever* been the weight you want to be? No, that doesn't include when you were a toddler or in fact at any pre-puberty age. I hate to break it to you but there are no short cuts, and by perpetually looking for them you are wasting valuable time.

It is, in many ways, about changing your mindset. Your success in the area of fitness and body image depends primarily on changing your attitude to it. Assume it is going to be hard, a bit mentally and physically painful, challenging on all sorts of levels and that it will involve some sacrifices, albeit only of the 'giving up the TV and sofa for an hour' variety. I'm afraid that in order to even *begin* to enjoy running and its numerous benefits, you have to commit to practising it regularly over a long period of time. It doesn't work any other way.

You must have a friend or work colleague or, at the very least, know of someone who is a running nut. Think about that person for a few minutes. Think of their physique and eating habits. Is the runner you are thinking of a total loser? Fat, lazy and woefully ineffectual at work? I didn't think so. Now ask yourself, are they fitter, more toned and healthier than you? Are they generally more positive, more proactive, more efficient operators? Does the runner tend to get things done, do what he or she says they are going to do, and exercise a certain discipline in other areas of their life? Do they seem to be able to get more done with less fuss? If, as I suspect, the answer to at least some of these questions is yes, running is the reason why.

```
To: The Grit Doctor

From: Nicola

Re: Small Win After Small Win

Every day was a different run. But the one
constant through it all was that for the first
twelve minutes of every run I just wanted to
stop. I would rather be doing anything else.
As I pulled on my socks at 6 a.m. in the dark
```

or during the first few metres on the pavement or when my lungs filled with cold air and said, 'Oh no, not this again', I would be wishing I was back in bed, at work, on the beach, in the pub, out with friends, playing sport, reading a book, watching TV — anything but this. My knees saying, 'Really?', my hamstrings tightening, my mind telling me to walk and the sensation that everything was about to break with a massive ping.

And then, as if out of nowhere, I would introduce myself to myself. My breathing would regulate, my muscles soften and warm, my heart would beat and chime 'good morning', my feet would find a rhythm and I would feel, see, hear and BE my body. And this happened every day I ran. Every day I would overcome the obstacle of myself — my motivation, my physical ailments — and win. Every day I ran I would win. Even if it was a bad run, it was a bad run out of the way — which was a win.

After a while this gives you such

confidence — a new and positive outlook. You train yourself that you will overcome any obstacle if you put the effort in. Small win after small win, day after day. If you put the effort in you win. No matter what happens during the day or what you have to face — if you run you win. I started taking that into other areas of my life. Things got done in areas where they hadn't been done before. More time was given to quality work, daunting tasks didn't seem so daunting so I was able to prioritise very effectively.

So my body became my body, the more I ran the more it became mine. It slimmed down, it strengthened, it shed excess, it felt good and it craved good things. I ate differently as my body demanded it — a diet I had never eaten before, a healthy diet, and I kept hydrated. My skin changed — softer, clearer. But the food was the major transformation. Good fuel food 80% of the time and then 20% of the time I ate and enjoyed whatever I wanted and it didn't matter.

Mentally I was clearer. I would leave the office with a jumble of thoughts from the day and over the period of my run home the irrelevant ones were stripped away and I was left with the important things to focus on. Problems would get solved so the stress would disappear and I would be left with what was important — invariably my husband and children.

THE GRIT DOCTOR SAYS:

There is an obvious connection between lack of motivation to exercise and general disarray in other areas of your life. This is every runner's secret: running is the key to successful living. By successful I simply mean living your life the way you choose to and being able to enjoy it fully.

MAKE RUNNING YOUR RELIGION

It is the practice of running that enables the rest of the runner's life to progress that much more effectively. Just speak to your runner friend and listen to them bang on about how their life has changed since they took up running. And anyone who has run a marathon will tell you that it really does take you to a whole new level of being and operational efficiency. In order to have the body you want you need to make running your religion. It is, in fact, much like the practice of religion in that it is *only* in the practising of it that you receive its benefits. Knowing about it and doing it once or twice will reveal nothing to you. It is only through a committed routine over several weeks and months that the benefits become evident – slowly and surely. You will see improvements not just physically, but in every area of your life. And it lasts forever or for as long as you choose to continue to practise.

Ruth

One thing that has struck me during the process of writing this book is how private running is for a lot of people. I wanted lots of case studies to inspire your good selves, so I emailed loads of friends who are keen runners asking for various opinions and stories to illustrate ideas in the text. Being runners, most were very efficient in getting back to me and all waxed lyrical about the incredible benefits of running to their overall well-being. However, many asked to remain anonymous. Now, it may be something to do with wanting to distance themselves from my book . . . especially as they all knew the title! But with a little bit of probing a few things became apparent.

1) Some people consider running to be their secret weapon in life and want to keep it that way – secret. It gives them an edge over all their non-running contemporaries that is so significant they don't want to share it.

2) Runners are perceived to be a bit 'square'.

3) Some runners are embarrassed by how cheesy the benefits of running sound and don't want to embarrass themselves or be seen to sound uncool. This makes me possibly the un-coolest woman on the planet, which causes me a considerable degree of pain and anxiety.

So, what to do with these interesting nuggets? I think that keeping things secret is a very good thing to begin with. It's all about letting your actions do all the talking. Declaring you are a runner when you are a bit overweight and not yet a practised convert operating like a well-oiled machine in all the other areas of your life could make you sound like a bit of a loser and also puts unnecessary and unhelpful pressure on yourself. Speak to yourself about it – a lot – but steer clear from announcing what you are doing until you have transformed your body and mind through the committed practice of running. My feeling is that people who talk about what they are doing before they have actually done it often don't live up to the promise. Be quiet and effective, actions speak louder than words and results speak for themselves. **Be a runner, don't talk about being one.**

THE GRIT DOCTOR'S GUARANTEE:

The Programme	The Results
No wasting money	Weight-loss
No recording weight	Fitness
No fitness checks	Better Health
No heart rate/blood pressure measurements	Increased pulling power
No faffing	Increased success at work
No frills	Confidence
No nonsense	Happiness

Ruth

My husband Olly and I were lucky enough to take a three-month honeymoon – the final stop of which was Perth, so I could meet Olly's totally gorgeous grandmother, then aged ninety-three. Olly adored his grandmother and it was very easy to see why when I met her for the first time. She clasped my face in her hands and said, 'Well, hello dear, I've been dying to meet you,' and sat me down for a nice cup of tea – the first of many.

It was Christmas 2009 and we were coming to the end of our trip, but we had spent only a fraction of the money we had saved, such was the generosity and hospitality of Olly's family and friends in Australia. Throughout our trip Olly had been talking about this novel that he'd had in his head for the past decade, he had practically written it the way he spoke about it – he had all the characters' names and the locations for the story, the entire plot and even the title. He seemed so keen to at least try to get this book onto the page. And so, in a moment of madness on New Year's Eve, we decided to resign from our jobs and take a further six months off to enable Olly to have a crack at writing. We posted our resignation letters on New Year's Day and then phoned our parents. Needless to say our 'plan' went down like something resembling a shit sandwich, especially when it was followed, a few weeks later, with the news that we were expecting twins.

We suddenly had this huge stretch of time in front of us and felt incredibly excited at the prospect of all the travelling we had left to do. The book would get written while we moved from place to place in South East Asia, the idea being that it would be the best place to travel on what was now a very tight budget. But it turned out to be very difficult to write when we were moving around from country to country and hostel to hostel – Olly became adamant that he needed to be settled in one place for his creative juices to flow. Fair enough, I thought. Plus I was desperate by now for some sort of settled routine and was dying to eat some of my own homecooked food. It was with all this in mind, that from an internet café in Laos we happened upon France (the food was the deciding factor) and sent numerous emails to owners of gîtes. One was out of our 600 euro a month maximum budget but looked so gorgeous – a bastide village house – that for a punt I emailed the owners. I told them we couldn't afford the advertised rent but that we could commit to four months and that my husband was writing a novel. The wonderful couple took pity on us and wrote back saying we could have it for 600 euro and that there was a lovely peaceful terrace and not one but two desks at which Olly could write. The airport was near enough with cheap Ryan Air flights for me to get back to the UK if and when necessary. Clearly this was meant to be.

I was in heaven when we arrived and I saw our kitchen — a huge farmhouse-style affair complete with all mod cons. My pregnancy cravings soon turned to pastry and all things French. Olly had brought an old copy of Larousse Gastronomique with us in the hope I would become some sort of Michelin-starred chef. I did learn a few tricks as I ploughed my way through it and have, I like to think, perfected the art of the tarte tatin and the soufflé. The idea was that I was going to paint and cook while Olly wrote. So far, so good. But it wasn't long before we started to struggle. I had done about one pathetic sketch since arrival and asking Olly for his word count was like poking a bear with a stick. And with each passing day, fewer and fewer words got written.

I kept thinking that if Olly would just run he would be able to write so much more easily. And that is how this book was born. Olly finally did what I had been telling him to do ever since we met: he put on his trainers, went outside and found himself a running circuit.

I make it sound easy when it was anything but. Poor Olly was very unfit and I knew he was going to hate the walking, get bored, run too quickly and get all puffed-out, then moan about it when he got home and probably never go again. So I briefed him on how to approach it — slowly, slowly, slowly. He did, to a certain extent, follow my instructions and at least he didn't overdo it so much that he did himself an injury or put himself off for life. Not during his first few forays outside anyway.

Bear in mind this is a man who has never failed to use any opportunity to slag off running with verve ever since we met two years before: 'It's so boring', 'I've always hated it', 'I don't know why you bother', 'I can't think of anything I'd rather do less'. I certainly had my work cut out for me to get him going and try to keep him motivated. I hasten to add that he did not do this for me or for the book. I swear, after two years of watching how I eat and keep fit, and listening to me drone on about where he was going wrong, he just woke up one morning and announced he was going for a run. I nearly fell off my chair. (He probably just went to get an hour's peace and quiet away from me but, hey, whatever gets you out of the front door.) He also told me to stop banging on about it and write it all down instead. So here I am. It is nothing short of a miracle. I truly believe that if he can do it, anyone can. And if I can convert him, I can convert anybody. Including you.

To: The Grit Doctor

From: Olly

Re: My First Run

The first five minutes felt pretty good. It was nearly all downhill, following the road out of our little village and down towards the valley floor; and with the wind in my hair, my belly giving me some momentum, and my legs finally starting to loosen up, I was beginning to think this might not be as bad as I'd feared. Then I hit the flat. Suddenly it didn't feel quite so straightforward any more.

After about five minutes of gentle jogging, I slowed, slowed some more, and then came to a halt. But Ruth's advice kept ringing in my ears so I forced myself to keep walking, even if it was with my hands on my head while sucking in air. I then walked for about the next fifteen to twenty minutes, until breaking into another

gentle jog. It didn't last long, and I
quickly reverted to walking again. I tried
very hard to appreciate the winter
landscape around me; the leafless trees,
the mud-brown fields, the fact that I
wasn't at work. At the end of the circuit
was a long section uphill back into the
walled, bastide town. I walked the whole
way up (hoping Ruth wasn't spying on me
from some unseen position) until I hit the
village square and then ran from there
back to our house. It was all of about two
hundred metres. I beat my hands on the
door, sweat dripping down my face, until
Ruth opened up and I fell inside. I felt
bloody terrible. All in all I reckon I'd
run about a tenth of the circuit, and all
of that downhill. I checked my belly just to
see if it had decreased in size. There was a
long, long way to go.

2

DELUSIONS OF *THINNEUR*

Running *improves your sex-life . . .*

As an aid to your sex life, there is no doubt that running improves the blood flow to those vital organs, giving you more energy and enthusiasm, if you get my drift. And if you are not getting any, running is a fantastic sex substitute – not only does the glow make you look as though you are getting plenty of action, but your more relaxed and calm demeanour is more akin to a woman who is happy and content (getting some) than the wound-up, tense types about whom people always say, 'She needs a good shag'. You know who you are.

RE-ACQUAINTING YOURSELF WITH YOUR INNER BITCH

The majority of us delude ourselves that we look a bit better than we actually do. A bit thinner; a bit prettier. We hold our stomachs in in front of the mirror, preening, pouting and posing in such a way that shows us in our very best light. Minus the double chin. With cheekbones. Our 'mirror pose' bears no resemblance to how we actually appear to other people. We never display ourselves like that when walking about, at work talking to colleagues or flirting in a bar. Occasionally you might catch yourself in a mirror unawares, or a shop window, and recoil in horror at the stooped, tired, cheekbone-less crone staring back at you. But you glance away quickly and stop off at the newsagents on the way home for a bottle of wine and a king-sized Snickers. Sound familiar?

HOME TRUTHS FROM THE GRIT DOCTOR:
Stop telling yourself that you look great when plainly you do not. You are robbing yourself of vital fuel required to kick-start you into action.

Try letting it all hang out, double chin included. Scrutinise yourself naked and tell yourself the ugly truth. In the quest for a better, leaner body, it is better to really make yourself *feel* fat and ugly. Do the maths: if you tell yourself all the time you are looking good, you are actually denying yourself the catalyst required to shift the fat from those body parts in the most dire need of improvement.

NEGATIVE AFFIRMATIONS

When my little sister was trying to lose a few pounds for a party and came to me for advice, it was with a degree of trepidation that I revealed to her my deepest, darkest weight-loss secret. When I want to lose a few pounds urgently, I look in the mirror early in the morning – pre-shower, no make-up and with my entire naked body in view – and I repeat to myself, over and over again, 'You fat bitch'. I then glance immediately at Cameron Diaz or another equally buff celeb in a bikini (*Grazia* magazine's illuminating celeb bikini-body specials are perfect for this part of the exercise) and the mantra begins to take on a life of its own. My sister laughed a little anxiously at this apparently demented pearl of sisterly wisdom. 'Try it out,' I said, 'and I bet your diet and exercise plan will be a great deal easier to follow. When you are tempted by something naughty for lunch, recall the images to mind – you vs Diaz – and repeat the mantra over and over again. I guarantee you will change your mind and go for the healthy option, and less of it.'

To: The Grit Doctor

From: Anna

Re: Are You Mad?

When my sister gave me this dark and
twisted advice to help me lose a few
pounds for a party, my initial reaction
was absolute horror. Firstly, wasn't Ruth
meant to say, without hesitation, that I
didn't need to lose any weight whatsoever?
Secondly, isn't this sort of thing
'thinspiration' and very unhealthy?
Thirdly, rather than calling myself a 'fat
bitch', wasn't I meant to love my body
blah blah blah? Anyway, knowing that my
older sister can be slightly unorthodox,
but as ever trusting her judgement, I did
as I was told. I found a picture of
Cameron Diaz running along the beach in
her stringy white bikini — athletic, lean,
happy and healthy — and I stuck it on my
bathroom mirror. Every morning when I got
out of the shower, I stood naked in front

of the mirror, looked at my body, looked at Cameron's, looked back at mine and said to myself (out loud to make it more punchy — again on Ruth's advice), 'YOU FAT BITCH!'

I don't really know exactly what it achieved psychologically, but it certainly made not having a morning croissant a lot easier. Thinking to myself, 'YOU FAT BITCH' and then averting my eyes as I went past the patisserie on my morning walk to the station had me giggling to myself. When I went out running I would think of Cameron bounding down the beach and the image would spur me on.

Sure enough, by the time the party came around I felt fabulous. Loads of people commented that I looked great, and my best friend even said, 'Anna, you're making me feel like a fat bitch!' I found myself giggling once more as it hit me: there I was at the party — lean, happy and healthy and feeling on top of the world.

As The Grit Doctor made clear from the outset, it's all about channelling your inner bitch. Don't have one? Yes, you do. It's simply hidden under layer upon layer of namby-pamby, self-delusional, positive rubbish which, luckily, is very easy to peel away. Here's how.

HOW TO CHANNEL YOUR INNER BITCH

Believe me when I say that we all have an inner bitch – in fact, I'd go so far as to argue that it's one of the things that makes us human. I bet you find it easy enough to tap into your nasty side when it's directed against others, don't you? Well, I want you to turn that judgemental, sharp-tongued bitch on yourself.

Close your eyes and take a deep breath. Bring to mind someone from work or a family member who really gets on your nerves. Focus on the specific quality or action that most incenses you about that person. Pause and contemplate the words and phrases that are now springing to mind quite effortlessly. *Voilà!* This is your nasty side. Congratulations. Isn't it amazing how loudly and clearly you can hear that voice when it is directed at others? OK, good. The key now is to turn your inner bitch against yourself. Say all those horrible things that sprung to mind moments ago, but this time *to yourself, about yourself.* Yes, YOU.

Now think about the part of your body that you dislike the most. Really dwell on it for a few moments. Then think of a celebrity who is lucky enough to be in possession of the perfect example of that very body part.* Imagine kidnapping the celebrity and stealing their thighs/arse/toned upper arms for yourself. Thy inner bitch shall covet Pippa Middleton's arse.

A GRIT DOCTOR HEALTH WARNING:

Keep your sense of humour at all times.

Next time you're sitting on the sofa, watching some banal reality television programme that you promised yourself you *would not watch tonight* so you could begin a new book/mow the lawn/clear out your wardrobe, just pause and listen carefully for a moment. Can you hear a nagging little voice, like a mosquito buzzing around in your head? 'Loser, I knew you wouldn't do it. I knew you would give

---

*And remember, only a tiny proportion of the picture-perfect Hollywood A-list are the kind of genetic freaks who are actually born with a perfect set of coltish pins or pert derrière. They pay their own Grit Doctor-esque trainers to work them into submission. And they don't eat. And don't get me started on what is done to your average celeb before you see her on the front of your favourite magazine: hours (possibly days) spent in hair and make-up before a photoshoot, only for the one shot plucked from the billion taken to get airbrushed to within an inch of its life. However, hot celebrities still look pretty good in the flesh *and* the mirror, so don't let all this cheer you up too much.

up, I knew you would fail. No one is going to believe a word you say if you can't even stick to a small promise like not watching this rubbish.' BINGO. That is your inner bitch.

Now that you have located that voice, you need to start becoming closer friends with it. Simply listen to it more often and imagine what it would say in certain situations. Answering for your inner bitch is the best exercise for strengthening your relationship. You are identifying and cultivating your nasty side and directing it against yourself to help you achieve success. The idea is not that you berate yourself to the point where the only reasonable response is to say, 'I'm so depressed I want to bury myself in a mountain of crisps.' It should be more, 'I am disgusted by this and I am going to do something about it right now!' There is a clear distinction between the two. Be bold and assertive in the language you use, not wimpy and victim-esque. Remember, the point is to get you motivated to run, not to binge-eat yourself to death.

If you are struggling to locate your inner bitch, try this visualisation technique: close your eyes and take a deep breath. Imagine a terrifying bitch you sort-of admire in real life (your old sports teacher from school perhaps) or a fantasy bitch (Meryl Streep from *The Devil Wears Prada* is a good one) and have a pretend conversation with her. What would *she* say if she walked into your sitting room now and saw you slumped on the sofa?

A GRIT DOCTOR HEALTH WARNING:

Remember that this is a DEVICE to help you get running and losing weight. Your inner bitch is not there to savage your self-esteem. Negative affirmations are not for the faint-hearted or psychologically fragile. If you are the kind of person who falls apart when criticised, this is not for you. You need to have a wicked sense of humour and be made of relatively stern stuff. The Grit Doctor does not want you to suffer a nervous breakdown in your quest to get fit and lose weight. So get some grit or get going.

Ruth

I honestly find 'negative affirmations' much more effective than their saccharine counterparts when it comes to getting me going. I think it's mainly because they make me laugh, although having said that, I always found the idea of 'positive affirmations' pretty amusing. Looking in the mirror and repeating, 'I am beautiful and clean and pure and I deserve to be loved', or some other such nonsense – I could never take myself seriously. In fact, is it ever possible to take yourself seriously when you're talking to your reflection in a mirror? The whole thing is just so unnatural. So if I'm going to do it, I find that calling myself nasty names is far more motivating and it has the added benefit of really making me laugh.

Humour is a great motivational tool – taking yourself too seriously can be paralysing and I experience a huge release when I laugh at myself. We all automatically feel psychologically lighter when we laugh and that somehow makes it easier to do things. That is my experience and I realise that perhaps it's not for everyone, but my sister and I have conversations along these lines all the time and never fail to cheer each other up. And I'm sure we're not the only sisters who are brutally honest with each other. If one of us is really down about something, whether it be putting on weight, a sudden breakout of horrible spots or some other dramatic life crisis, the other never takes a softly-softly approach. It's much more likely to be along the lines of, 'Yes, you are a fat bitch – sort it out!' which instantly makes the other laugh and start to feel better and, crucially, motivated. In facing your fears, sharing them and having them confirmed, rather than batted away by a well-meaning friend – 'No, you're not fat! You're curvy!' – you are bravely facing up to the truth. This allows you to do something about whatever it is that's making you *unhappy. The minute a friend tells you what they think you want to hear, you go straight back to the sofa and your* Mad Men *boxset, happily devour a tub of* Phish Food *and remain safe in the knowledge that you're not fat, you're basically Christina Hendrick's doppelgänger. (You're not. She's curvy. You are fat.) But if you take matters in hand and run an 8-miler on a Sunday morning, you can eat that ice cream without a trace of guilt and probably pull Don Draper afterwards.*

It is, of course, very dangerous to start really beating up on yourself, but I believe you really have to be ill already or very fragile for this method to cause you any real harm. The key to it all is a cracking sense of humour. The test is if this hasn't made you laugh so far, it's probably not for you!

SEVEN KILLER EXCUSES

1. I don't have the right build for running

There is no such thing as the right build for running. Any build will do. This excuse hides an underlying fear of failure. Large-breasted ladies, in particular, are fond of this excuse. Well, I ran a race with a double-E cup lady friend. She wore 2 sports bras and had less nipple-chafing than I did (a B cup on a good day) *and* she beat me.

To: The Grit Doctor

From: Alice

Re: Being Supportive

I didn't think I had the right frame for
running. I had what is referred to as a
'heavy frame' supporting an overly large
chest that had been known to cause more
than one person to walk into a lamppost and
many more to talk to my chest as if it had
a personality of its own. Running was not
comfortable. As a teenager, I wore two
swimsuits to avoid unwanted buoyancy when
swimming. So, in my early thirties when I
took up running, I wore two bras to avoid
the bounce. It worked on that front but did
nothing to divert the crass comments. But I
continued running and although plugging
into music didn't drown out the running
commentary on my chest ('Release the
animals' was a memorable cat call ...) I
perfected the art of the vacant stare past
the culprits. Sports bra technology has

improved over time and so the extra bra is no longer necessary. And although two pregnancies and age mean my chest has been unflatteringly described by my children as 'long', continued running means it has actually shrunk a little and people are now more likely to talk directly to my face. Plus, through running (and now triathlons, too) I feel good about my body for the first time and no longer care what other people say or think about it.

2. I hate running

Good. You would be a bit of a freak if you didn't. Everyone hates it until they have practised it religiously for some time. Hating something shouldn't stop you from giving it a go. Hate and love are a hair's breadth away from each other – you know the cliché. So, if you hate it (and with vitriol, like my husband) you are in fact in a very strong position. You have passion, and once you take it up, you will love running at least as much as you once professed to hate it.

3. I couldn't run at school, it's so boring

No, being fat is boring and, worse, whingeing about being fat and doing nothing about it is more boring still. Don't you remember that most things were boring when you were at school? Being young, for example. Remember how much you wanted to be a grown-up and have a job? Couldn't have got that one more wrong now, could you? We are not at school any more so get over it. Immediately.

THE GRIT DOCTOR SAYS:
Our excuse-making machinery is in-built and poisonous. Regular attacks by your inner bitch will help tear it down.

---

4. I don't have the time

My personal pet hate. Everyone has the same twenty-four hours a day. How do you think President Obama finds the time to go on his daily run? Do you think he conjures some extra time out of thin air? No. He has the same twenty-four hours as you, and I guarantee he has more to get done in any given day than you probably do in an entire week, and I mean a really busy week. Get over this one quickly. Get up earlier. Go to bed later. Or get organised and run to and/or from work. The latter option would most likely eat into the least amount of your time, if at all. Running is the least time-consuming of all sporting activities.

5. I need to do 'X' first

This is 'I don't have time' in disguise. It is the excuse that, on some subconscious level, is stopping you from attempting stuff that challenges you. Accept that you can always tell yourself there is something else you need to do first. But this is just white noise. Ignore it.

6. It's raining; it's too cold; it's too dark; it's too windy

We live in one of the worst climates for rain. But look at it this way, neither the FA Cup Final nor the London Marathon get cancelled because of the rain. Rain is no impediment whatsoever to a run. In many ways it is a bonus feature. There is nothing quite like the feeling you get if you stick two fingers up to the worst of the elements and just run. The world rewards you for your efforts by making you look ten times rosier than after a run in less arduous conditions and leaves you feeling like you could climb Everest. Dress appropriately and go for it. I promise you, when you have done this once you will never use the weather excuse again.

As for 'it's too dark' ... well, don't be a wimp. Running in the dark is great. Especially if you are at the beginning of this programme and are feeling shy about being seen as you venture out for the first time. The dark doesn't stop you getting to the pub and back or from finding your way home from a dodgy nightclub in the wee hours. The only thing to remember is that you must take sensible precautions, most of which are blindingly obvious but just to be on the safe side I have listed them in Appendix 1: Health and Safety.

7. I can't do it

Yes. You. Can. (Repeat this to yourself over and over again in the style of President Obama for maximum effectiveness.) And in the next chapter, The Six-Step Programme, The Grit Doctor will show you how. You don't need a better body and you don't need to get fitter first. You don't need more time. *You are ready for this exactly as you are.* You just need to read for a few more minutes and then get up off the sofa and out of your front door. It is as simple as that.

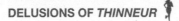

THE GRIT DOCTOR SAYS:

Either do this thing or don't, but don't disempower yourself by making up excuses all the time. It is boring and makes you weak. Choose 'yes' or 'no' and cut out the rubbish in-between. So, take a deep breath, shut out all the white noise in your head and turn the page.

3

THE SIX-STEP PROGRAMME

Running makes you feel less deranged . . .
There is a truly meditative quality to running that for me is a most cherished benefit. If I am anxious or afraid or just unbelievably stressed, nothing will cure me better than a good hour's running. Better still, if you are already feeling fantastic, going for a run can almost be hypnotising. Everybody's experience is different but all runners will know exactly what I am talking about. This morning Olly reported feeling incredibly peaceful and contemplative during a run: 'Sometimes my head becomes completely empty and I am able to think about nothing.' This is a wonderful position to be in – freeing your brain up for anything or nothing.

So, here we are. With luck, your sense of humour is still intact and you are feeling pumped about getting started. In six simple steps and over the course of eight weeks, I am going to teach you how to run. Follow the steps and **don't skip any**. You will need to use your common sense and be sensible about your limits.

THE GRIT DOCTOR SAYS:

Adapt this programme to suit your own weight and fitness level without any fuss.

I am keenly aware that getting started may be the hardest part for you, and there is, of course, the all-consuming embarrassment factor. The 'buts', the 'ifs', the 'stuff' that stops you from getting off your arse and out of the front door. You buy the kit, you make promises to yourself and your other half and you venture out once, only to give up, utterly humiliated that you were completely puffed-out after ten minutes. This will not happen ever again if you follow The Grit Doctor's simple Six-Step Programme. Because **anyone** of **any size** and **any age** can do this.

FAST TRACKERS observe the six steps and get cracking. SLOW COACHES read the six steps and then follow the detailed programme in chapter 4.

STEP 1: YOU ARE ON YOUR OWN

Drink a large glass of water. Wearing comfortable clothing and a pair of trainers (don't buy new ones for the occasion – anything reasonably supportive will do at this stage), leave your front door and head out on foot for your nearest green space. If you have no access to a green space, walk through the streets near your home. **The aim of Step 1 is to walk out of your front door and create a loop which starts and ends at home. This will ultimately become your running circuit**. Wear a watch if you like so that you can time the whole outing, but there is no need to be over-precise about it. You want it to take roughly an hour and a half door-to-door, which should work out to around 3 or 4 miles. Ideally the circuit wants to be relatively flat, some-where you find interesting and pretty is a great bonus, and as little concrete as possible, to spare your joints. But it must be a circuit – not several laps around the same park – just one continuous circuit home, ideally not covering the same ground twice.

Walk the circuit at a comfortable pace. Unless you are very unfit, you should be able to walk the circuit easily. If you are struggling, just slow down, but try not to stop. Speed up your walking pace if you fancy it and feel com-fortable. OK, well done. You've established a circuit, and you've walked it without stopping. This is a great beginning.

THE GRIT DOCTOR SAYS:

Do this first circuit on your own. It is hard enough motivating yourself without the added burden of having to motivate someone else too. A problem shared is, in this case, a problem doubled. At this stage a friend will make everything much harder. Their broken engagements, pathetic excuses and negative, dispiriting chat will hold you back. 'It's not working, let's join that Pilates class instead', 'Ooh, let's have a milkshake, it won't kill us'. It will. You can of course introduce a newcomer to the practice and share with them what you have learnt, and indeed run with them, but **only once you have 'got it' yourself**. Step 1 is not the time to rope in a mate. This is about you, not anyone else.

STEP 2: WAX ON, WAX OFF

Repeat Step 1. Double check with yourself that you really do like your circuit: that you enjoy the scenery; that it is long enough (minimum 1.5 hours walking door-to-door); that you are not intimidated by the other people you come across; that it isn't dangerous; that you won't get lost. Is there any way in which you would like to alter it, improve upon it or lengthen it? If so, make the adjustments now. Are your clothes comfortable? Are you wearing a good supportive bra? Are your trainers comfortable? You're not too hot? Not too cold? Good.

STEP 3: DO NOT RUN BEFORE YOU CAN WALK

Repeat Step 2. Now walk it again tomorrow. And the next day. Walk it a bit faster each time or bits of it a bit faster each time. After a few days or weeks, depending on your starting weight and fitness level (which The Grit Doctor expects you to assess for yourself), you should be building up your strength and walking it more quickly and easily. You should be feeling confident about your route, and relaxed because you are beginning to know it backwards.

Don't be completely thrown by the idea of assessing your own fitness level. This does not mean you should get sidetracked by spending money on having your fitness assessed at a gym or getting your 'fat ratio' or heart rate measured, or any other such fiddly thing. Just look in the mirror and have an honest conversation about where you are at fitness-wise. How many weeks or decades has it been since you last did any exercise? (And that **doesn't mean** a dash to the bus stop or kicking a ball about in the garden.) What does your body actually look like? Can you see any muscle or is everything buried under layers of flab? Be honest and realistic. **Even if you have done no exercise at all EVER and are extremely fat, you can still do this programme**.

THE GRIT DOCTOR SAYS:

If you can winch yourself out of bed or off the sofa, and make it to work or to the shops, you are fit enough to start Step 1.

Remember there is **no running until walking your circuit has become second nature**, i.e. you can do it easily without becoming breathless and you feel totally ready – body and soul – to break into a slow jog. You will gain confidence about when you are ready to make the transition because your breathing will have improved considerably since your first outing, when the walk may have made you feel breathless. Plus, if you have been completely sedentary for some time, the weight will probably have started to come off just from the walking which should be incredibly inspiring and help motivate you to continue.

If you are slim, don't be fooled into thinking you are necessarily any fitter than the fatties. You can be very slim indeed and still incredibly unfit. For you skinnies who have done no exercise whatsoever, do the walk and see how you get on. THE BREATH TEST is an excellent way to determine what you are capable of. You should always be able to hold a conversation while walking fast and jogging slowly. If you cannot speak or say a sentence you are overdoing it. Likewise, if you can sing the national anthem, crank it up a gear.

THE GRIT DOCTOR'S RECAP:

The only fitness test to bother with is THE BREATH TEST – the most fuss-free test known to man.

STEP 4: SLOWLY, SLOWLY, CATCHY MONKEY

OK, you are now ready to start running. Set out for your walk as you did in Steps 1, 2 and 3. After walking at a brisk pace for about ten minutes to warm up, allow yourself to break into the slowest sort of run you can imagine. The difference between a fast walk and a very slow jog is this: when a fast walk turns into a slow jog, you bounce up and down a bit as your feet lift off the ground (no matter how slowly you jog, *you should always bounce*). The slow jog should follow on totally naturally from the pace of your fast walk. Break into this *very slow jog* and resist the urge to speed up. You will run out of steam too quickly. Go slow. Go slower. As slowly as is humanly possible. The aim is to go as slowly as you can for as long as you can without having to stop. As soon as you have to stop it is time to walk, not to sit down, and certainly not to collapse on a park bench with your head between your knees praying that you don't have a heart attack. What I am saying here is that it's very important that you never stop moving. Got it? Good.

So, now you gently 'run-walk' through your circuit, ideally every day but four or five times a week is fine, gradually building up the distance that you run before you start walking again. The best way is to build on this from the same spot each day, trying to lengthen the distance you can jog before you walk the rest of it. Yes, you can break into another small trot later on after walking, but in order to measure your progress effectively, it's best to start from the same place and extend it, even if it's only by a few metres each day or five minutes each week.

Ruth

This routine was born when I moved back home for a year to live with my mother – then fifty-seven years old. I was thirty and keen to clear the last of my student debt. (It had cost me thirty thousand pounds to become a barrister – insane career choice. Do not do it.) So, Mum kindly took me in. Now, I know how she feels about me. She loves me dearly and is very proud. But she also finds me a bit hectic, a bit full-on and a bit of a 'food-fascist', if you will. You see Mum is a very relaxed and happy soul, so I know it was with a degree of trepidation that she accepted me back into the fold.

After I had ruthlessly spring cleaned the kitchen – the fridge and all its contents, and all the cupboards – we finally sat down to a nice cup of tea and a natter. It was then that Mum revealed that she was keen to get fit and lose weight. She had enjoyed an active sports life right through her forties, playing netball to competition standard. She is also Catholic (this is a huge advantage, both for getting in touch with your inner bitch and for self-imposed grit of any kind). But at fifty-seven she was flagging. Without much energy, she was a bit down in the dumps about her weight and possibly a little bit lonely with Dad working abroad a lot of the time. I could barely contain my glee. What a wonderful project for me: to become my own mother's personal trainer and live-in dictator.

For Mum, the circuit was a lap around our local parkland, Virginia Water (or Vag Waters as we call it). It is about a 3.5-mile circuit. Mum was convinced she couldn't do this. That she was too fat, too old, too embarrassed. She had never run long-distance before (although had enjoyed hurdling in her youth). We started out just walking it. Marching, swinging our arms, nattering the whole way round. Then we started oh so very, very, slowly running, and I mean at a snail's pace, the first stretch of the circuit. Each day she extended the running stretch by a little bit and before long (about two months later) she was able to run round the whole circuit very slowly, no problem. She was so chuffed with herself.

This was five years ago. She still does that circuit but has added regular gym visits and swimming to her repertoire. She may still have the odd toffee, but she also eats a lot more fish and green veg. She is no longer under any illusions as she is in touch with her inner bitch and has the voice of The Grit Doctor ringing in her ears whenever she tucks into a scone. That hour around Vag Waters gave her back her confidence and sparkle and more importantly gave her so much more energy to put into the rest of her life. Oh yes, and she lost loads of weight. But you know what? After a while you forget about the weight-loss. It becomes merely an incidental bonus and no longer your reason for running.

To: The Grit Doctor

From: Mum

Re: The Truth About Running

I played netball and squash after I had my four children and stayed quite fit until my early forties. But I hadn't done any exercise, really, for the last fifteen years and certainly not since going through the menopause. I was missing it, but honestly thought those days were over for me.

When Ruth came home I was impressed by her committed approach to running and healthy eating, and noticed how much calmer and contented she was after a run. Whenever she was in a bad mood, I would tell her to go running! I wished I could go with her sometimes, but knew I could never run as I was too old and too fat. Luckily Ruth had other ideas. She took me on as a sort of project I think, determined that I could run and I must say she was a very kind and persuasive coach.

I didn't get special shoes or a special bra, but we went to Virginia Water and walked round it. It is about 4 miles, I think. It's a lovely walk by a lake and we chatted all the way. Ruth told me to walk briskly, swinging my arms as we went. After a few times just walking round she told me to jog with her for a bit, which I did. We did it so slowly it felt a bit silly but I still got quite tired, quite quickly. She sensed this and told me to stop and walk the rest of the circuit. We probably only jogged for a minute that first time but she congratulated me at the end and I felt as though I had really achieved something. Each time we went I jogged a little further. It was easy to improve each day because I would try and jog to a tree or to the bench just beyond the tree or to the swans just beyond that — always pushing myself the smallest amount further.

One day I made it all the way to the half-way point around the lake. I couldn't believe I could get that far. I was thrilled and realised it wouldn't be long before I could go the whole way round. The first time I did I wasn't just pleased with myself, I was amazed. I told anyone who'd listen! I started doing it every day as I enjoyed it so much.

I always jogged very, very slowly but when I finished I was hot and felt like I had done a lot of exercise. Ruth assured me I'd lose weight easily even at my age and it really did just fall off, despite my rather bad eating habits. And I was so much happier in myself. Getting up in the mornings for Mass, doing the shopping and even the ironing — which I can't stand — seemed easier. I knew it was the running so I just stuck with it.

> I must confess I hadn't run round Vag
> Waters for a while when Ruth told me
> about the book — I had been going to the
> gym instead and running on a treadmill —
> but since I read the book I've got right
> back into it ... mainly because I am
> terrified of The Grit Doctor!

STEP 5: KEEP WAXING

Repeat Step 4 consistently. Stretch yourself little by little each time, until you have completed the circuit by running all the way from start to finish (excluding the walking warm-up) without stopping. You will be so proud of yourself. By the time you do the entire circuit, you will be totally ready for it, having built up your stamina slowly and steadily at a rate suitable to your fitness level. You have given yourself the best present ever. And it'll stay with you for the rest of your life. All you need to do is keep it up. Three times a week is the minimum, five times the optimum. The run should take you roughly forty-five minutes door to door, and anything up to an hour is great.

To: The Grit Doctor

From: Olly

Re: Yes I Can

It was about six weeks after my first run
that I finally completed my circuit without
walking. It felt completely amazing. In
the week leading up to it, I'd almost done
it on a few occasions only to be foiled
both times by the final steep slope up from
the valley floor to the town square. A day
or so later, I tried again, but this time,
for whatever reason, I didn't even get
close and ended up walking for the whole
of the last fifteen minutes. It was
incredibly frustrating. I had a day off
after that, and it turned out to be a good
idea, because it was during the following
day's run, fully refreshed, that I finally
cracked it.

I remember the feeling of triumph that
spread through my body on the uphill

climb when I suddenly knew I was going to make it. I ended up sprinting the last few hundred metres like a madman, the blood pumping through my veins, my adrenalin through the roof, the *Rocky* theme tune playing in my head. It felt stupidly good, and I couldn't wait to tell someone about it in unnecessary detail. Unfortunately for Ruth, there was no escape.

A GRIT DOCTOR TIP:

Do not try and jazz things up by doing fancy warm-ups and stretches. You probably don't know how to do them properly anyway and doing them incorrectly will make you look like a proper loser. Walking briskly and swinging your arms is the perfect warm-up. Hold yourself up straight, and pull your stomach and arse in. Try and maintain good posture at all times while running. Warm down in an identical fashion at the end of your run.

STEP 6: GET ADDICTED

Repeat Step 5 three to five times per week, week after week, month after month, until you can't remember a time when you didn't do it. **Let it become who you are as opposed to something you do**. Get addicted. Sometimes treat yourself to a longer run. Go off-piste. Go somewhere totally new. But only when you have really built up your confidence. Other runners will smile and nod knowingly in your direction. They too are in the club and may have been for many years. They are welcoming you in.

```
To: The Grit Doctor

From: Nicola

Re: Long Run, Short Run, Hot Run, Cold Run

Every day was a different run: short run,
long run, fast run, slow run, jog and
walk, sprint and jog, medium-distance
slow, short-distance fast, cold run, warm
run, hot run, good run, bad run. It all
varied and I suppose that is when you
```

truly come to love something, the moment
you understand the subtleties that exist
within an activity that to everyone on
the outside looks exactly the same.

THE RUNNER'S REWARD

Now that you're a real runner, the time has come to indulge
yourself in a binge at your nearest specialist running shop.
My favourite is Run and Become in London, but there are
many fantastic specialist stores all across the UK, a few of
which are listed in Appendix 2. Now, be warned: the staff
(undoubtedly all supremely fit runners) and the bewildering
array of kit can be a tad intimidating for the novice. Have
some running chat and questions lined up ('I'm thinking of
entering a 10 km race – any good ones you know of?',
'Which bra would you recommend?') before you enter with
your head held high.

Once you are in, ignore all the kit and gadgets and focus
on the shoes. They are different, very different, from
normal trainers, even those trainers that claim to be running shoes. Do not fear the absurdly wide-ranging choice
of shoes on display. These shops work like magic. The
assistant will tell you which pair you need and indeed

which size you are. Believe it or not, you may not be the size you think for a properly fitting pair of running shoes. Take a ticket, like at the meat counter in a supermarket, and wait for your number to be called. Then simply say you want a pair of running shoes – and you can own up that it's your first pair – and before you know it you will be outside, running up and down under the watchful and highly trained eye of said assistant until they – not you – are satisfied that you have the right pair. This will set you back at least sixty quid. But it's the best sixty quid you'll ever spend. When you get home, put on your new shoes and take them out for a spin. Walking and running is going to feel so much better in these shoes. So different. So much easier. So much more comfortable. You will never ever want to run again in anything other than these perfect running shoes. Which is a very good thing because these shoes are your first line of defence against injury.

THE GRIT DOCTOR SAYS:

I am not one for frivolities, but this one piece of kit is an absolute wardrobe essential once you are a practising runner. Non-negotiable.

To: The Grit Doctor

From: Olly

Re: Shoes!

Back in England for a few days and as a
belated-birthday pressie, Ruth took me
along to Run and Become in Victoria to buy
me my first pair of running shoes. It was
time to cast aside the old tennis shoes
I'd been using since my first French run
and get into something new.

Ruth had prepared me for the fact that
this shop was a mecca of running, and she
wasn't wrong. It had a lot of shoes in a
very tight space. It also had a staff of
indecently thin men and women who looked
like they ran a marathon before breakfast.
One of them proceeded to ask me an amazing
number of questions about my feet and my
running. She then selected about three
pairs of trainers and made me run up and
down outside with them on to see which one

was the perfect fit. She wasn't just going to let me pick the first ones that felt OK. She wanted to find me the ones that would work in harmony with my running soul. And she did.

4

RUN WITH THE GRIT DOCTOR

Running makes you regular . . .
 If you suffer from constipation, running is the cure!

OK, the six steps are to be treated like the ten commandments – sacred and not to be argued or tampered with. For you Fast Trackers, the six steps alone will be sufficient. For those Slow Coaches amongst you, I have devised a day-by-day, eight-week programme to literally walk you through those first steps into running a full circuit. Anyone, and I mean *anyone*, can do this – it is based on my mother's journey from walking to being able to run a 3.5-mile circuit. I have allocated two rest days per week, but you can take a maximum of three and a minimum of one, and you can vary this from week to week.

If you find it helpful to keep a journal of your progress, there is a running log at the back of this book designed to work in tandem with the eight-week programme. Tear it out and stick it to your fridge if you think it will help you. But DO NOT be distracted by list making, record taking and general faffing.

THE GRIT DOCTOR SAYS:

The eight-week programme is to be undertaken while observing the six steps at the relevant times.

EIGHT-WEEK PROGRAMME

WEEK 1

Monday
Read Step 1, then plan yourself a suitable run that starts and ends at your front door (see Appendix 2 for mapping websites that can help with this). Remember you will be walking this. I recommend a 3–4 mile circuit. So plan it and then walk it. Go on then, but don't waste too much time on the internet. In fact, if you know this is a particular weakness of yours, don't map your run at all, just go outside, start walking and use your imagination.

Tuesday
Rest day.

THE GRIT DOCTOR SAYS:

No stuffing your face as a reward for yesterday's exertions. You do not deserve it.

Wednesday
Read Step 2. Repeat Monday's walk.

Thursday

Read Step 3. Repeat Monday's walk, but quicken your pace – swing those arms and march confidently round your circuit.

Friday

Rest day.

A GRIT DOCTOR REMINDER:

Rest days are not 'reward' days.

Saturday

Read Step 4. Begin as per Thursday, **walk the first ten minutes**, then break into the **very slow jog** described in detail in Step 4 and sustain for **five minutes**. Walk the remainder of the circuit.

Sunday

Repeat Saturday.

THE GRIT DOCTOR'S GUIDE TO ACHES AND PAINS:

In any committed exercise routine there will be aches and pains and the odd twinge. The Grit

Doctor expects you to tolerate these minor ailments and not to whinge about them incessantly to your other half. Under The Grit Doctor's tutelage, you should build up your muscle tone gradually and ought not to be in for any nasty surprises, but your muscles may feel tired to begin with, especially in the thighs and arse. Do not be put off by this and under no circumstances give up. Do not run out and purchase 'supports' either, unless you have a *real* injury. Just persevere and the side effects will reduce as your fitness level improves, and your muscles firm up and adjust to being used properly.

Wear your 'pain' with pride. This can actually be quite a pleasant feeling – the feeling of muscles having been worked on. Enjoy it. It is physical proof that you have pushed yourself outside your comfort zone: a badge of honour. Reflect with horror on how you have never felt anything in these places before and how inspiring it is that finally, after all this time, you are working those long-forgotten muscles. The odd stitch is no reason to worry either. Drink more water (don't neck a litre in one go just before setting out, just stay constantly hydrated at all times). Refer to the Health and Safety section at the end of the book for advice on how to prevent and what to do in the event of serious injury.

THE GRIT DOCTOR SAYS:

You absolutely must not skip an exercise session on the basis that you have got a stitch, or that your muscles ache. This is simply your excuse-making machinery at work trying to thwart your attempts to change. Ignore it and soldier on.

WEEK 2

Monday
Rest.

Tuesday
Repeat what you did at the weekend – I'm referring to the walk/run, not the drinking binge.

Wednesday
Repeat Tuesday but extend the jogging part to **ten minutes** *and slow it down*. Walk the remainder of the circuit.

Thursday
Repeat Wednesday.

Friday
Rest.

Saturday
Repeat Thursday.

Sunday
Repeat Saturday.

DISTINGUISHING BETWEEN GOOD PAIN AND BAD

Do not run with a temperature, if you are vomiting or if you have diarrhoea (this should be patently obvious), and be sure to wait until you are fully recovered before getting back into running, as your body needs all its energy reserves to stave off any infection. If real illness strikes, you may need to go back a week or two in your running plan to re-build your strength and stamina. Be sensible about it. If you have spent a month in intensive care recovering from malaria, be sure to take things really slowly and do a lot of walking before you attempt to run again. If, however, it was just a twenty-four-hour bout of food (or alcohol) poisoning, that shouldn't set you back more than one day's training – just make sure you are properly hydrated before you set out.

THE GRIT DOCTOR SAYS:

A common cold is no excuse to put your feet
up. If you've only got the snivels, a run is not
going to kill you, in fact, it might make you feel
a lot better. But take it easy at first, and know
your limits. Be responsible for your body and let
common sense prevail.

WEEK 3

Start with a **ten-minute walk** to warm up, followed by **fifteen minutes' incredibly slow jogging**, followed by walking
for the remainder of the circuit without stopping. Two rest
days of your choice, but not consecutive to one another.

THE GRIT DOCTOR SAYS:

Nothing in this life of any value is gained
without pain and sacrifice.

WEEK 4

Ten-minute walk to warm up, followed by **twenty minutes' jogging** (slow down the pace of the jog if necessary to

86

sustain it for twenty minutes), followed by walking the remainder of the circuit without stopping. Two rest days, but not on consecutive days.

WEEK 5

Ten-minute walk to warm up, followed by **twenty-five minutes' jogging** (slowing down where necessary to avoid stopping altogether), followed by walking the remainder of the circuit without stopping. Two rest days as per previous weeks.

THE GRIT DOCTOR SAYS:

It does not matter how slowly you jog, remember the aim is to sustain your movement, either the jogging or the walking part, for the entire circuit without stopping. Keep slowing down.

WEEK 6

Ten-minute walk to warm up, followed by **thirty minutes' very slow jogging**, followed by walking the remainder of the circuit without stopping. Two rest days.

WEEK 7

Ten-minute walk to warm up, followed by **thirty-five minutes' very slow jogging**, followed by walking the remainder of the circuit – there may be almost nothing of it left! Two rest days.

WEEK 8

Ten-minute walk to warm up, followed by **forty minutes' very slow jogging**, followed by walking home if there is anything left of the circuit – if not, always warm down those muscles by walking a few hundred metres before you go back indoors – it's the ideal warm-down. Two rest days. **Read and observe Step 5**.

THE GRIT DOCTOR SAYS:

Once you are able to complete the circuit, then and *only then* should you start to increase your speed as your fitness level improves. The sky is now the limit.

WHAT NOW?

Read and observe Step 6. Take time to congratulate yourself and really acknowledge your achievement ... and OK, that's enough. Consolidation is now key: absorbing your running routine into your weekly schedule and making it stick to you like glue. This bit is going to be easier than you think – you got over getting started and that was the hardest part of all. Everything else is easy in comparison with that because you have done it gradually over time and slowly assimilated the regular practice of running into your very being. You will notice all sorts of unexpected benefits – some instantly, some later on – and you won't want to give them up.

If you have a great deal of weight to lose, then an even bigger 'well done' to you because getting started was even harder due to the sheer physicality of carrying that extra weight through the circuit. So you deserve a huge pat on the back. No, not a cream cake. The weight will literally fall off. I promise you.

And no, you don't need your own special programme if you are fat, although if you are morbidly obese (go to your GP and ask), please seek medical advice before embarking on any kind of fitness programme. I'm confident that any doctor would wholeheartedly endorse you strapping on a pair of trainers and getting moving, albeit slowly. To be brutally frank, if you are morbidly obese, you won't be able to manage anything more than moving very slowly anyway until some of the excess weight has shifted. You need to really focus on getting moving. NOW.

PUT YOUR FAITH IN A HIGHER POWER: THE RUNNING-SHOP ASSISTANT

After a while, you'll start to notice that those shiny new trainers you bought yourself are looking a bit tatty – usually after about 350–500 miles of running. (That sounds like a hell of a lot, but if you're running 4 miles, four times a week, you *could* get through a pair of trainers in around thirty weeks.) So, it's time to head back to your local specialist running shop. This is like your graduation. Armed with your battered pair of trainers, you will take them back to the assistant and bang on about how you wore them out running 'NYC' (or your local 5 km race). The assistant will be immediately recognisable to you as the same toned runner who sold you your first pair of proper trainers (and therefore something of a goddess) but she, however, won't have a clue who you are as you are about half the size you were when you first went into the shop. Don't embarrass yourself here. She has been running for decades. Maintain an air of laid-back cool. You may think it's the greatest achievement in the world to have run in a race, but at these kind of shops people eat marathons for breakfast. So, you will return the shoes battered and worn to the assistant, who will inspect them and then choose you a new pair, most probably the very same shoe in an updated model. I love this process. That you don't get to choose, that the assistant decides. Like God. You put your trust in her. And she always gets it right.

THE GRIT DOCTOR SAYS:

The Grit Doctor does not approve of 'runners' with special water bottles and straws coming out of rucksacks, with stuff attached to their arms and stopwatches and all that. But as long as you don't let it detract from the thing itself – that's the run, in case you've forgotten – then anything goes. And incidentally, you don't need to drink throughout a 4-mile run provided you keep hydrated at all times during the day and drink plenty of water afterwards. But buy and wear as much kit as you like, especially if you find it motivates you. After all, it takes all sorts to make a world.

Ruth

I've been running now for ten years and have had some wonderful (and some awful) experiences. Training for the

London Marathon was, as you know, my first foray into
running. The race itself was and extraordinary. I seemed to
experience every single emotion that I have ever felt while
running it: from complete despair to hope; anxiety, fear and
pain to incomparable joy. Totally weird and unexpected. I
was moved to tears by a complete stranger who had
terminal cancer but ran miles 23–25 by my side and
prevented me from stopping. And I was moved to tears of
another kind at the finish, this time frustration, by failing
to overtake Frank Bruno (who seemed totally out of
condition to me) and a guy with NO LEGS. Yep, I was
beaten by a man with no legs.

But my greatest, or perhaps I should say most memorable,
marathon experience was in New York. My old friend, Jane,
was running this one too and I was determined to beat
her after the humiliation of my earlier defeat. I like to
think I would have done but for the fact that I had
promised (practically by way of a blood oath) to look
after my flatmate who I had trained to run it and whose
entire family had flown out to watch. Her father had
made me swear not to leave her side throughout the run
and I was true to my word.

Jane had taken it upon herself to bring a mobile phone,
camera and a banana to the start line. I looked at her and
thought how silly she was to be so encumbered at the start

of the marathon . . . and then she asked me to carry the banana for her. She then prised the support from my gammy knee and slid it on to her own leg, much to flatmate's escalating distress. Why did I say yes to either of these requests, you may ask? Where was The Grit Doctor? Well, the truth is, I owed both girls . . . big time. For some reason we'd been really constipated since arriving in New York and the night before the race I insisted we all take laxatives to sort ourselves out. I practically forced everyone to take double the dose to ensure it worked. This turned out to be a very BIG mistake. The next day we were all suffering from crippling tummy pains and had not got off the loo all morning. I was entirely to blame and so lending a knee bandage and carrying a banana seemed a small trifle in comparison.

My flatmate wanted to go super slow which was fair enough. Jane did not so abandoned us pretty early on – also fair enough. What was perhaps not fair enough was when my flatmate decided to go so slowly she was, in fact, walking and I had to run backwards and forwards to keep myself going and be true to my promise not to abandon her. Five and a half hours later, we crossed the finish line, really running now and holding hands. It was very moving – I hope for both of us. The best thing though was the food we ate after the race. Flatmate's wonderful family took us to this fabulous restaurant where the portions were enormous (although, I am reliably told, paltry in comparison with the rest of America – note to self: must run marathon in another American state to sample portion size) and we devoured about three cows' worth of ribs like scavenging dogs. Meat had never tasted so good.

Towards the end of the race though I kept thinking, Next time, Ruth, you run for yourself. No people to look after and definitely no sharing of injury equipment. No carrying bananas, no artificial pace-setting by anyone else. That was eight years ago and sadly there has not yet been a next time. I really want to run one with my sister or my brother or my mum, or perhaps all four of us together, in a country we have not yet visited.

Five years ago, I went on holiday to Kenya with my sister. The Grit Doctor came with us, tightly packed into our suitcases. She leapt out the first morning at about 5 a.m., beckoning us down to the beach to go running. We had talked a lot about running on this holiday so it was in an almost holy silence that we put on our swimwear and a T-shirt, and tiptoed outside to take the short three-minute walk to the beach, where we started to run.

This was a 6-mile stretch of coastline, littered with hazards: some parts felt quite dangerous and there were areas where the sand was less smooth and bits where we were followed by slightly mangey-looking dogs. But by day three we had got our run nailed. The best thing about it was seeing all these young Kenyan men and children at the crack of dawn training on the beach, doing sit-ups and press-ups, sprints, interval training, or long-distance runs, and, without fail, one or two would join our run. When we got to the end, back to the resort, morning had broken and we dived into the sea in total ecstasy before tucking into an enormous breakfast buffet. My sister still teases me about how un-holidayish our holiday was on account of all the running (and reading) that took place, but I know she loved it and wherever she goes she is sure to run – it is the best way to make friends with a new environment and feel as relaxed and happy as you ought to on holiday. It also leads to guilt-free eating. I must say that we both came back from that holiday with a real glow.

I have still never been on a run with Olly – that is a great running memory for the future ... although in trying to outdo each other, I fear we may both do ourselves an injury.

PART 2

EATING

5

RUN YOURSELF THIN

Running helps you pull . . .

Before I got married, if I had a date on a Friday or Saturday night I always made sure that I went on a run beforehand. Not only did it calm my nerves and ensure I was on good form – relaxed, but chatty and genuinely happy – but also I knew I would be looking my absolute best.

You will be so chuffed with yourself for fitting in a run beforehand, and that translates into looking good. You won't have that horrid loss of appetite that mars many a good date either. Your date will find you miles more attractive if you order the burger and chips and actually manage to eat them. Plus, you won't need to down ten gin and tonics beforehand for Dutch courage; the run will give you all the courage you'll need. You will glow and you will enjoy yourself.

THE GRIT DOCTOR SAYS:

Part 1 of this book needs to be completed and
mastered before you can go on to make any of
the changes in Part 2. Running and the practice
of running are what your diet is all about. By all
means read on now, but ensure that you have
completed the Six-Step Programme in chapter 3
and are committed to running regularly before
even thinking about changing your eating
habits. Ignore The Grit Doctor at your peril.

I have a real problem with the word 'diet'. It is invariably
used to mean weight-loss. This is not what the word diet
really means – in fact, the online *Oxford English
Dictionary*'s primary definition is 'way of living or thinking', which seems to me to be a much healthier
interpretation of the word. But because you almost certainly associate 'diet' with punishing weight-loss regimes,
we're going to try to use a different word in its place
wherever possible: FOOD. Because you are not going on
a diet as you know it. You are running regularly and
losing weight. What you now need is the right fuel to
accommodate your new lifestyle and burgeoning appetite.
The great bonus is that you will want all this food anyway
because, through running, your body will be crying out

for it. In short, the hard part was getting you running. The food part is EASY.

FAT VERSUS THIN

Your past relationship with food and your current body shape will influence how you read this next section and what you take from it.

If you are **thin** and have no desire to change your weight at all, you still need to read Part 2 because it's possible you're not eating enough and you may not be eating the right sort of food to fuel your running addiction.

If you are **too thin**, or have eating issues of any description, you should **seek medical help**. Running and messing around with your eating patterns is not advisable if you have any underlying eating disorder. It can be dangerous to exercise and diet if you fall into this category and I do not want to be responsible for making your condition worse. TAKE RESPONSIBILITY FOR YOUR BODY AND SEE YOUR DOCTOR.

If you are **fat**, you will lose weight quite effortlessly through running. But you probably have some bad eating habits which you should change in order to keep yourself fit, healthy and, crucially, able to continue running regularly.

If you are **very fat** or even morbidly obese and are not

losing enough weight through running and really struggling to run because of the excess weight **READ THIS SEC-TION VERY CAREFULLY INDEED**.

GRAVE AND WEIGHTY MATTERS

So how do you figure out the truth about your own body shape? Well, you've already done the naked mirror assessment and hopefully The Grit Doctor has forced you to confront your wobbly bits. But for the purposes of this next section, I recommend you weigh yourself *just once*. It is extraordinary how many women (and men) lie about their weight, as much to themselves as to others. The number of women who say, 'I'm about ten stone', when they are frankly closer to twelve, do other women a serious disservice. It's your real weight we want, please, *not* your fantasy weight. You are not the weight you were as a teenager when you last got on the scales at a compulsory school medical check. Just because you can still *squeeze* into the same pair of jeans you wore ten years ago does not mean that you are the same weight.

Go to a Boots store with a set of electronic scales which print out your weight and BMI. You can even work it out for yourself using an online calculator (try http://www.nhs.uk/Tools/Pages/Healthyweightcalculator.aspx), or for added grit factor, seek a professional medical opinion.

When you've got the results DO NOT try and cheer yourself up. Acknowledge the awful fat truth – it is extremely useful grist for your running mill and should have you back outside terrorising the streets before the day is out. (And be thankful that the weighing-in part of this book came *after* you started running, not before. Just think what the number could have been . . .)

THE GRIT DOCTOR'S ORDERS:

Do not buy yourself a set of scales. You will only waste valuable running time obsessively weighing yourself.

TARGET WEIGHT

Now that you know your real weight, identify your target weight. And this is where you put away the picture of the slender celeb you used to spur you on in your early runs. I'm talking about the ideal *healthy* weight for your age and height. *Do not create an unhealthy target weight inappropriate to your age and height.* DO NOT GUESS. Use the online calculator or ask your doctor. And always bear in mind, especially when you feel suicidal about how many pounds you still have to lose, that 90% of the work is already done.

I kid you not. Because 90% of your 'diet' is continuing to run three to five times every week. And each week, the pounds will continue to fall away.

STILL A FAT BITCH?

Most runners tend to be fairly healthy eaters because once you get fitter you naturally care more about what you put into your body, plus you need the right sort of fuel to run efficiently. Because you are happier, you will also be less inclined to eat away negative feelings, a vicious circle many overweight people get caught up in. Six months into your running programme, without any dramatic changes to your diet, and I reckon you will be well on your way to your target weight. But if you are really fat, and haven't a clue about good eating habits, or don't seem to be losing as much weight as I promised, it is because you are eating too much of the wrong foods.

This section on food is going to be short. Dieting, diets and talk of them are extremely boring topics. Remember that the beauty of running is that not only does it make adopting new and better practices in other areas of your life so much easier, but *it*, the run, will also act as your 'diet'.

I hope that you are already at the point where you *want* to eat more healthily. It is a weird side effect of running. And so when this does happen, The Grit Doctor wants to be there to help you make good food choices. That is what this section is about. IT IS NOT ABOUT DIETING. THERE IS NO DIET. YOUR RUN IS YOUR DIET.

Once you get into your running routine and experience a surge in appetite, it pays to stock up on the 'right' foods and acquire some good habits in order to accommodate your raging hunger. If you are relatively healthy anyway, with no nasty eating habits, then you genuinely do not need to change a thing. Just stick to the **two golden rules** which follow and continue running. *The weight will fall off.* You can really enjoy your food and not worry about making any drastic changes. However, if you are regularly eating foods on The Seven Deadly Sins list (page 120) then you are filling yourself up with rubbish and useless calories. This will make running more difficult and your weight-loss less dramatic. You need to be healthy to be a practising runner and you need good fuel for your body. But you don't ever need to skimp on portion sizes or deprive yourself of a treat (or indeed the odd blowout, indulgent calorie-fest) because it is running that is keeping you thin, not your food choices. If you are training for a marathon and using the plan in Part 4 of this book, you need to up your intake of carbs to fuel your training. There is advice on this, and recipes, in Part 4.

If you feel that you are really fat and need to make some drastic changes to the way you eat, then I suggest you follow the ideas in this section very carefully. You probably know what it is that you need to stop eating and you know what you should be eating instead, but so far you have chosen to ignore the obvious. However, there is good news. You have transformed yourself into a runner and that brings with it an *automatic shift* in your attitude to your body and what you choose to put into it. Capitalise on this change of attitude and take advantage of the increased motivation you have developed through running, to tackle your food issues.

This is why it is so important to master the running first. It gives you the vital energy and motivation to assure your success on the food front. Whether you have the odd bit of tweaking to do, or a radical overhaul of your eating patterns, you will be able to confront this issue now much more effectively as a runner. So, what follows are the **two golden rules** and some tips to take on board, which will be nothing short of a pleasure for you, a committed runner in touch with her inner-bitch.

A GRIT DOCTOR REMINDER:

Running is the key to your weight-loss, not food.

6

THE TWO GOLDEN RULES

Running buys you time . . .

If I have something I really don't want to do (usually work-related), I know that if I go on a run first, I will be able to complete it more quickly and do a better job. Even though the run itself eats forty minutes into my evening, the work will be finished earlier than if I didn't go on the run. It is a very strange paradox. A run is an investment in time. So never think of it as time out, but as time multiplied.

1.

DRINK MORE WATER

2.

EAT
LESS
CRAP

7

DIETING DELUSIONS

Running gives you great legs . . .

Not only is it the ultimate calorie burner for all-round body improvement, it is the only exercise I have found that really tones those parts of a woman that are especially prone to sag – in particular, the thighs and bum. I'm convinced it banishes cellulite. Having good legs enables you to wear all sorts of clothes that you otherwise might shy away from post-thirty, like short shorts and mini-skirts, and to look really good in them.

1. I'LL START THE DIET TOMORROW

This is the main reason why you are unable to give up being fat. It is not about starting a diet. It is about changing some bad habits. And *right now* is the only time you've got. Pour yourself a glass of water, put a baked potato in the oven and make that the beginning. Next, throw out all your fat-laden foods and treats. Exorcise your cupboards and fridge and give them a good spring clean. Go to the shops, on foot if you can, and stock up on all things good for you. Do this now, and it will be a very strong beginning because as we already know, *getting started is the hardest part of all.*

It is really important to bin the whole concept of dieting in your quest for a fitter, healthier and slimmer you. I cannot re-iterate enough the importance of GIVING UP DIETS. And while you're at it, give up starting stuff tomorrow. Begin it now. Whatever it is. DO IT NOW.

THE GRIT DOCTOR SAYS:

Dieting is a dirty word. It is never about slavishly following a diet. It is about changing habits, shifting attitudes and taking responsibility for your body.

---

2. I'LL START EXERCISING ONCE MY DIET WORKS

Wrong. As we've already discussed, it's *the other way round*. This bears repeating because it's a really dangerous concept which needs to be challenged. *You need to get running first in order to start feeling good about yourself.* It's only when this begins to happen that you will want to eat more healthily. Any dietary changes you need to make will actually be far easier to embrace once you are a committed runner, because a happier, fitter you is in a much stronger position to change. In fact, healthier eating habits will come quite naturally to you once you have established a good running routine.

THE GRIT DOCTOR SAYS:
DON'T GIVE UP. There is a permanent escape route from a life spent trapped in a fat body and running will help you find it.

---

3. I'M BIG BONED

Really? Are you? If you genuinely think this might be the case, get a professional opinion. Go to the doctor, get weighed and ask if you are overweight. You may be big boned, but you may also be fat. Being big boned is no excuse for being overweight. Chances are you are kidding yourself.

4. I DON'T LIKE VEGETABLES AND SALAD

Oh dear, spoilt as well as fat are you? You clearly didn't get thrashed for not eating your greens as a child. Bad luck. This whole thing is going to be a lot harder for you. Princesses can be very resistant to grit. But imagine how much you would impress others (others being people *other* than fellow princesses) if you were able somehow to change something about yourself. That you are reading this book is a very impressive beginning.

5. I DON'T LIKE WATER

I am not asking you to *like* water. I am telling you to drink it. There is a distinction between the two. I don't think to myself, 'Ooh yum, I'd love nothing more right now than another glass of tap water!' Nobody does. Water is essential fuel for all your bodily functions and upping your intake is fundamental to running safely and to the success of any long-term 'healthier you' plan. Herbal teas are fine and, if you must, sugar-free drinks, although this is only a last resort as they are full of junk and only keep you in the bad habit of craving or thinking you are craving something sweet all the time.

THE GRIT DOCTOR SAYS:

It depresses The Grit Doctor how something as simple as drinking more water is such a barrier for so many people. Really, what's wrong with you people? In place of water you drink fizzy drinks and endless cups of tea and coffee. Not only are these drinks full of useless calories, but most of them act as a diuretic, so they *de*hydrate rather than *re*hydrate, making you thirsty, tired and lacking in energy. For the love of God, drink more water.

---

6. I HAVE A REALLY SLOW METABOLISM

Bullshit. You are overweight because you eat too much of the wrong food.

8

THE GRIT DOCTOR'S PLAN FOR PERMANENT WEIGHT-LOSS

Running gets shitty jobs done . . .

No, not literally. But my God, it helps. Ironing. Washing-up. Dusting. Vacuuming. Supermarket shopping. Running makes all those deathly boring daily tasks easier to do. My theory is that because of the happy hormones that running stimulates, you become much better at 'getting on with life' without so much resistance and complaint. When it comes to domestic drudgery, a run is nature's very own equivalent to 'mother's little helper'. Everything is easier to bear after a run. Consequently, you get everything done much more quickly and efficiently.

THE SEVEN DEADLY SINS

1. **Fizzy drinks** are crack cocaine without the weight-loss benefits. They have no place in the fridge. Not even the diet ones which are also filthy and disgusting and make your breath stink. Do everyone a favour and give them up. The only fizzy drink you should ever consider consuming is water. And champagne.

2. **Sweets** are for children and have no place in an adult's life. Grow up. Give them up.

3. No more **snacking** on . . .

4. **Crisps**, **cakes** and **biscuits**.

5. **Pastry** is dangerous. Delicious and dangerous. I feel strongly about this, partly because it seemed to be an essential part of my daily pregnancy needs and wow did it pile on the pounds. Remind yourself that pastry is basically butter: totally delicious, flaky buttery heaven. Anything that tastes that good is going to be bad for you. If you do cave in to temptation and eat it, be sure to enjoy a punishing run that day and tell yourself over and over again and in no uncertain terms that you are indeed a FAT B!TCH. This should help to prevent a relapse.

6. **Fast food** and . . .

7. **Takeaways**, The Grit Doctor's bête noire. Not only are they incredibly fattening and nutritionally redundant, they encourage the sort of couch-potato living that you are trying to reject.

THE GRIT DOCTOR SAYS:

If you are consuming any of the above as part of your daily diet, this is the reason you are not losing as much weight as you would expect to from running alone. Frankly, as an adult you should be ashamed of yourself if you are still buying sweets and fizzy drinks on a weekly basis. Stop it now.

The Grit Doctor's Orders:

- Eat only three meals a day and eat them AT MEAL-TIMES.

- Eat your evening meal EARLY.

- Eat slowly and chew thoroughly. As with running, SLOW DOWN.

- Eat SMALLER PORTIONS, especially of the bad stuff.

- Load up your plate with VEGETABLES, preferably green ones. Ideally, half of your plate at mealtimes should be made up of vegetables.

- Use LESS OIL AND FAT in cooking and spread butter thinly. Be really anal about this.

- CUT DOWN ON PUDDINGS. They are not a daily staple, but a treat. Fresh fruit and natural yoghurt are exceptions to this rule.

AND, LEST YOU FORGET:

- Make RUNNING 3–5 times a week a habit. Get it into your head that your run is your diet.

- Drink water. DRINK MORE WATER.

THE GRIT DOCTOR SAYS:

There is so much nonsense out there about diets and weight-loss that it is very easy to get completely overloaded with advice (which is often useless) and embroiled in overly complicated food regimes. Do not get side-tracked by all the dieting information out there. It is all a complete waste of time and commits you to a very boring lifestyle. You can be slim and eat normally if you run at least three times a week.

9

GOOD FOODS

Running *gives you a flat stomach . . .*

During a run, think about your posture and use the run to improve it. Regular running will make you proud of your stomach – the flab will disappear while toning up the underlying muscles at the same time quite effortlessly.

For extra midriff tone, try and get into the habit of running while tensing your stomach muscles. Sound deranged? It is. Imagine your back in the position it should be in if you were doing a sit-up correctly – the small of your back should be pressed into the floor – and try to recreate this posture while running. It is not easy and I often forget to do it myself, but at the very least, get into the habit of holding your stomach in and lengthening your torso while you run.

What follows are just some examples of 'good' foods that you should introduce in a big way into your diet. It is by no means an exhaustive list. If you are at your target weight, you are hopefully already eating the right foods. If you are the wrong weight, sit up and pay close attention.

- **Pasta and bread**. Yes, those very foods which are often the ones most diets tell you to give up, should be eaten by the shed-load. HOO-bloody-RAY. Unless you are wheat and flour intolerant, **bread and pasta are the absolute staples of the runner**. Eat them without a trace of guilt. It is the butter and sauces and jams and cheese that we lather on top of them that make them fattening, not the pasta and bread themselves. Obviously brown bread is better than white. But more importantly, spread your butter *really* thinly. At all times. Scrape off any excess bits. Every little knob counts. It is, after all, pure fat.

- **Potatoes**. Another thing they say you should give up on a 'diet'. I beg to differ. A baked potato is another perfect food for the committed runner. Prick with a fork, wash in cold water, then dry thoroughly. Rub salt into the skin and bake away – a great thing to put in the oven before you go out running to devour upon your return, all crispy on the outside and creamily fluffy on the inside. Mashed up with some cheese, butter (remember the rules) and **baked beans** they can't be beaten.

- **Raw vegetables**. As already stated, you should make green your favourite colour. When it comes to vegetables, remember that the closer they are to raw the better. Steam or lightly boil them to retain their goodness. Keep raw veg in the fridge for snacking – carrots, cucumber, peppers etc. You will need plenty of healthy snacks at the ready to accommodate your increased appetite.

- **Lean red meat**. Perfect for replenishing iron stores and much-needed protein.

- **Fish**. Obviously. Not only fresh fish, which can be expensive, but tinned sardines, mackerel or tuna on wholemeal toast or a bagel are fantastically nutritious.

- **Wholegrain cereals and porridge**. Ideal fuel for running. Eat with skimmed or semi-skimmed milk. Or water if you are in the mood for self-flagellation.

- **Chocolate** can be eaten IN MODERATION. It is not normal to eat a bar of chocolate every day as part of your lunch, but it is a great energy boost and treat before, after, or indeed, during a run (just ask Paula Radcliffe).

- **Fresh fruit and yoghurt**. Stock up on these for snack attacks.

- **Dried fruit and nuts, Ryvita, crisp breads and the like**. Ditto.

THE GRIT DOCTOR SAYS:

Trying to find low-fat versions of your favourite junk foods (low-fat crisps, low-fat chocolate bars, low-fat or sugar-free biscuits) is FATAL. It only serves to keep you trapped in your bad habits, such as having a packet of crisps with your lunch. It is still a bad habit, even when disguised as a low-calorie/low-fat/ low-sugar alternative, and is more often than not packed full of rubbish ingredients. The idea is to get out of the old bad habits and into forming new good ones. Raw veg, fruit, or yoghurt are what you want to train your brain to be craving at lunch, not a packet of crisps.

10

THE GRIT DOCTOR
KITCHEN CONTROL

Running helps you sleep . . .

This was a massive and unexpected bonus for me when I took up running. I experienced once again the sort of teenage and pre-teenage sleeping scenarios which I had long since forgotten: going out like a light when my head hit the pillow and not only that but into a deep and satisfying sleep. Heaven. None of that staying awake for ages with thoughts and anxieties racing through my head. A good run on any given day almost certainly guarantees a good night's sleep thereafter.

THE GRIT DOCTOR SAYS:

Take control of your eating habits. Start cooking
your meals from scratch using fresh ingredients.
No more slavishly following the latest diet fad or
hot new chef. You are in control now and you
need to start thinking for yourself.

And before you object with the 'I don't have time' excuse, or
'I can't afford it', this is fast and economy cooking at its best.
You need to get back in touch with what it is that you are putting into your body and begin to exercise the same discipline
over your kitchen as you are exercising over your running.

A GRIT DOCTOR TIP:

Don't go overboard in following any eating
regime. The rules are there to be broken every
once in a while, provided you are running at
least 3–5 times a week. Indeed, you can break
them regularly *once you have reached your
target weight.* The Grit Doctor wants you to
take responsibility for your weight and your
body without becoming some sort of hairy-
armpitted, birdseed-munching health freak.

I am not a chef and this is not a cook book, but there are a couple of basic staples that every runner should have in their culinary arsenal. Quick, nutritious and TASTY, they are also brilliant for any of you who suffer those guilt-ridden *God-I-really-ought-to-cook-my-children-something-from-scratch-like-Jamie-does* moments. The key is to learn a few simple bases you can cook without even having to think about the ingredients, quantities or method. Then you can get as creative as you want to, jazzing them up as the mood takes you. It's a bit like mastering your basic running route before you start going 'off road'.

PASTA

As we've already discovered, pasta is the runner's friend. But sauce and cheese are not. The key with any type of pasta sauce is 'less is more' – less sauce means you can eat more pasta. Crushed raw garlic and thinly sliced chilli stirred through piping hot *al dente* spaghetti with a drizzle (not a gallon) of olive oil, chopped herbs (parsley or basil always work), seasoning and grated parmesan (on the thinnest part of the grater so you use the least amount of cheese) is a delicious and filling meal, not to mention incredibly quick and easy to prepare.

To this great base you can add any number of other

ingredients. Or try some of the recipes in Chapter 20, although bear in mind that these are designed for marathon runners, so adjust quantities accordingly.

Before long you will have developed your very own repertoire of pasta supper recipes – fuss-free and delicious.

SOUPS

Again, get the base right and you can create and develop your own recipes. Sweat a chopped onion with finely diced celery (garlic is optional) in a little oil and butter (listen for the voice of The Grit Doctor when you're adding in fats). Then add your vegetables, cut roughly into bite-sized chunks, and sweat until softened. Next, add chicken or vegetable stock (fresh is best but a cube will do) and simmer very gently for a maximum of twenty minutes. Don't boil it to death or you will lose all the goodness from the veggies. Blitz with a hand-held blender, in the Magimix or indeed mash with your potato masher if you don't have the kit or just love added grit factor. Continue until you have the consistency you like. Add more boiling water to thin if necessary. Parsley is a great herb for flavouring soups at the end and extremely good for you, being high in calcium and vitamin C.

Make a big batch as your soup will keep in the fridge for

up to three days and provides you with an ideal lunch after a good run. You can also freeze batches in individual portions to help organise your eating.

THE GRIT DOCTOR SAYS:

If you have a long-standing weight problem and are trying to lose weight, it is a good idea to plan your meals at the beginning of the day or even for the entire week, leaving less room for excuses or possible meltdowns. This is why it helps to have frozen batches of soup and other healthy meals at the ready. Keep mealtimes and choices simple and uncomplicated.

STIR-FRY

Get a wok. The stir-fry is another Grit Doctor staple. It is unbelievably quick to prepare and the method of cooking ensures the vegetables retain all their goodness.

Use the tiniest amount of oil and heat for a minute on a very high heat. Then throw in a chopped onion, finely chopped chilli, garlic and ginger, and then add prawns or diced chicken, beef, or pork (as lean as you can) and stir-fry for a good five minutes. Then chuck in some raw vegetables for a couple of minutes. Keep stirring. Add some cooked noodles or rice at the last minute and a splash of soy sauce if that's your thing. *Voilà*: instant, healthy goodness.

THE GRIT DOCTOR SAYS:

Steer clear of all ready-made sauces and 'easy-use' garlic, stock and so on – they are invariably full of junk and hidden calories. Fresh, raw ingredients are the key. Easy on the fat and meat, heavy on the vegetables and noodles or rice.

RISOTTO

I love a risotto and always make one the evening after having a roast chicken to make use of the delicious fresh chicken stock and remaining pieces of meat from the carcass. It is one of Olly's favourite suppers.

For the base, fry a chopped onion in a smidgen of butter. Cook until soft and translucent. Add the risotto rice and stir for a few seconds, ensuring you coat all the rice in the onion and butter. If you want, you can add a splash of wine at this point but it's by no means obligatory. Then add the chicken stock, boiled, ladleful by ladleful until the rice is cooked but still retains a bit of firmness. Reduce the heat and add some finely grated parmesan. If you have good chicken stock this is a delicious meal without any extras.

If you do want to add a bit of razzle-dazzle to it, try adding diced, cooked veggies such as leeks or asparagus. Or you can stir through raw spinach or rocket leaves, or meat, if you have any knocking around.

Risotto isn't the fastest meal to prepare, but I cheat and add half the stock immediately on a low heat, keep my eye on it and stir it occasionally rather than constantly as you are supposed to.

FRUIT SALAD

Make up a big bowl of fresh fruit salad at the beginning of the week. Fruit is much more inviting when all chopped up and colourful, and ready to eat in a big bowl staring out at you every time you open the fridge. Add a splash of fresh orange or apple juice to the mix and then you can tuck into a bowl whenever hunger strikes and only something sweet will do. Add some freshly grated ginger for added zing. Or eat with a dollop of Greek yoghurt (but *not* the whole carton).

JUICE

If you're seriously committed to increasing your intake of fruit, I thoroughly recommend getting a juicer.

Try one of the following recipes:

- Juice two carrots, one apple, one orange and 1 oz ginger

- Two carrots, one apple, one kiwi and a handful of parsley

- Two apples, half a beetroot, half a cucumber and a handful of fresh spinach

- One tomato, two carrots, a celery stick, basil and the juice of half a lemon

All are totally delicious and put you well on your way to your five a day. And you can even add vodka on a Friday night for a tasty and nutritious cocktail.

THE GRIT DOCTOR SAYS:
It's about having the right foods ready and accessible and not having access to the wrong ones. It is very difficult even for The Grit Doctor to resist the pull of a Chocolate

HobNob when the packet is staring out from the cupboard. It wouldn't be an issue if there was only a packet of Ryvita on offer. If you are trying to lose weight, don't have both in the cupboard. Don't cripple yourself with choice.

SMOOTHIES

I perfected the art of the smoothie while in France. I had the luxury of a Magimix there, but a hand-held blender is also ideal for the task. I bought stacks of frozen raspberries, strawberries, and other summer berries which had the twin advantages of being cheap and of making the smoothie ice cold.

The base of a great smoothie is banana. To this, add any number of other ingredients. For dairy-free, fruit-only smoothies add some fruit juice – orange or apple is ideal but really any juice will do, the purpose is to make the smoothie into a drinkable consistency. Then in go your frozen berries, any number of fresh fruits, or a combination of both. Experiment. I discovered tinned pineapples are a fantastic ingredient (those in juice not syrup). For a real treat, add a small pot of vanilla yoghurt.

A GRIT DOCTOR REMINDER:

It's all about knowing what makes up the 'base' of things. Armed with a good base, you can develop your own recipes to suit your taste preferences and budget, and start adapting meals to what you have left in the fridge rather than being tied to a list of obscure ingredients all the time. A good base and the right cooking methods are the foundation stones upon which to develop your culinary skills.

A LITTLE SOMETHING EXTRA FOR THE SEASONED SADO-MASOCHIST

Allow yourself to feel real hunger pangs. These may be entirely alien sensations to you. The general advice with any sort of dieting is, of course, the complete opposite, namely: don't allow yourself to get hungry and keep your sugar levels up. And no doubt there is a sound basis for this – if you allow yourself to feel really hungry, you are more likely to cave in and binge on sugary rubbish. However, as a disciplined runner, you are no longer so weak-willed. You are stronger and more determined than the rest. Let yourself feel real hunger pangs and learn to appreciate them.

Learn to recognise when you are *really* hungry, as opposed to just bored, tired or sad.

Let the feeling last for as long as you feel comfortable and then eat healthily. Don't give yourself any other option. Don't have fatty foods at home. Don't have sugary treats stocked up in cupboards. Remember, your treat is losing weight through running. Whenever you are tempted to snack or binge on forbidden foods, first look in the mirror, summon your inner bitch and repeat the immortal phrase, 'YOU FAT BITCH'. And before you eat anything, drink two glasses of water. You may find that you are not in fact hungry at all.

THE GRIT DOCTOR SAYS:
Hunger is often thirst (FOR WATER) in disguise.

But The Grit Doctor *also* says:
There is another kind of thirst that water cannot quench. Alcohol is fine in moderation. The aim is to work hard and play hard and look good at all times. The odd blowout session on a Friday night is to be recommended. The Grit Doctor does not want you to live like a saint. The idea is to get running so that you can enjoy the rest of your life more fully – food, fun and Friday-night sessions included.

RUNNING ON EMPTY

Running on an empty stomach first thing in the morning is a truly phenomenal experience, especially if you can time it so you run through the sunrise. Keep your clothes and shoes and everything you'll need ready by your bed the night before, so you can literally roll out of bed and get into them while still half-asleep. The only other thing you need to do is drink some water and you are ready to go. **No faffing**.

If you are anything like me, you will not feel remotely hungry before or during this run. You will instead feel as light as a feather and be able to run so much more easily than at any other time during the day or evening. Nothing sets you up for the day ahead in quite the same way. It will leave you feeling euphoric, unbelievably relaxed and content, but also incredibly effective and razor sharp.

A GRIT DOCTOR TIP:
Running on empty isn't for everyone but try it and see before making up your mind.

Running will fundamentally change your relationship with food. You can run on empty and not feel hungry for up to an hour afterwards. But when you do feel hungry, you will be ravenous. Soon after a run is the best time to eat, especially if you are trying to lose weight. Your metabolism is at its peak after a run, blood pumping hard through your body, everything working smoothly and efficiently, so you burn off what you eat quickly and easily, much more so than if you had eaten before the run and tried to use it to burn off the calories. Eating before your run will also make it far less enjoyable, as you will feel very heavy and sluggish making the whole experience feel like more of a trial. So, try and run first thing in the morning on an empty stomach if at all possible. Don't panic if you can't, it doesn't matter. I used to run before supper in the evenings (on an empty stomach) and that worked well for me too. The morning run is the absolute ideal, with the beach run at sunrise being the mother lode. Do it when you next go on holiday and write me a thank you note.

THE GRIT DOCTOR SAYS:

If you are overweight you are almost certainly eating to fill a hole that is not always about hunger. No amount of food is going to fill it. A run will.

PART 3

NOW WHAT?

11

MOTIVATION MELTDOWN

Running makes you pretty . . .

When I was pregnant and enjoying that much-fabled 'glow', my skin looked remarkably similar to how it used to after a run. It makes perfect sense. When pregnant, your blood supply increases and blood is much closer to the surface of your skin, contributing to that healthy glow. After a run you glow too, because your blood is pumping a lot faster around your body and the capillaries close to the surface of your skin become dilated. And to glow is to be at your most beautiful. Run your way into a glowing complexion, plumped out skin, and rose-tinted cheeks. This is probably the most effective beauty tip you'll ever be given. No amount of make-up, facials, surgery even, can match the look of your face after a run.

So now you need to turn everything you've learnt into a habit. But how? Keep doing it over and over again. Wax on, wax off. You are exchanging your old bad habits for new good ones. Beat yourself up when you mess up – be really hard on yourself. The idea is that once your new running and eating regimes become habit – and they will after months of repetition – they won't go away. They will become part of who you are and how you operate. And you will no longer have to think about them or motivate yourself to do them. They will just happen quite naturally as part of your daily routine. I'm talking about running, drinking more water and taking responsibility for what you put into your body.

Repeating the identical, tried-and-tested run, day in, day out, is precisely the sort of boring habit you need to cultivate in order to guard against motivation meltdown. The more routine the run is, the more effortless it is to do, until eventually it becomes another part of your day that you no longer have to think about. You will just do it – like washing and eating – and you won't be derailed by outside forces. The more simple and uncomplicated you make it, the easier it will be to cultivate and coax your run into becoming a habit. It becomes more like sleeping and less like going on a date – fraught with decisions and choices about what to wear, where to go and what to talk about. The lower the choice factor, the greater the chance of simply doing the thing without thinking about it or trying to worm your way out of it. Yes, it's robotic – that is precisely the idea – but you won't be complaining when you have the body you always dreamed of and can still eat like a king.

MOTIVATION MELTDOWN

It happens. You let down your guard and your motivation suddenly leaves you completely. This is the only real hurdle you will come across in your quest for success – you will wake up knowing that you have to go for a run today and you won't want to go. You will keep putting it off: 'I'll go after lunch', 'I'll go this afternoon', 'I'll go when I've watched X'. The irony being that you won't be able to enjoy X or be productive with the rest of your day until you go on your run. The guilt will grind you down, distracting you from being effective elsewhere.

This guilt is a very important tool to help you get back outside. Because if you miss the odd run, the guilt gets to you and will probably force you back into your trainers the next day or later that week. But when the odd day turns into a couple of months, then you are in real trouble. The guilt will fade and you are in danger of forgetting everything you have learnt. Your running memory is very short where motivation is concerned. The inner bitch that pesters you when you are running regularly is silenced through lack of use. And once she is silenced you have lost a valuable motivational aid. That voice is your own personal trainer. Keep her talking and she will get you into your trainers and back outside.

At the risk of repeating myself, this is why it pays to have a set routine for when you go running each day: with a strict routine you can't start playing these pointless mind games with yourself. Your run shouldn't be one of any number of possible options for you to choose to do on any given day, but an ingrained part of your daily routine. When motivation meltdown strikes, be hard on yourself. With a sense of humour, do the 'YOU FAT B!TCH' routine in the mirror, and you should be back outside smiling in no time at all.

The beauty of running is that even if you fall off the wagon – and no matter how long you stay off it – you will still only ever be two minutes away from having it back in your life again. It doesn't require any re-training or any new extra commitment. However, depending on how long you were established in your running routine beforehand, you may require a gentle re-introduction. If you hadn't even completed the Six-Step Programme for example, and fell off the wagon for a fortnight, then definitely go back a week or two. Know your limits and be realistic: if you only did a few weeks of the programme and then took a gap year, you've got to start again from scratch.

THE GRIT DOCTOR SAYS:

To get back on the wagon, all you need are your running shoes and the courage to take those first steps outside.

BE GOAL-CENTRIC

Transform motivation meltdown into motivation zeal by paying to enter a race and pledging to raise a sum of money for charity, ideally one that is of great personal significance. And tell everyone. That way you won't be able to wriggle out of training. Setting yourself goals and putting yourself out there – whether it's a race to achieve your personal best, raise money or beat a friend – is guaranteed to keep you motivated. Check out the internet and join a club if that's your thing (see resource section at the end of the book) – or run against a work colleague and beat them. It's all about setting yourself targets, and winning.

THE GRIT DOCTOR SAYS:

Anyone who thinks of running as 'fun' does not know the meaning of the word. At school, running is a punishment alongside detention and lines, for God's sake. It is not meant to be fun. If you try and make it fun you will fail. Fun is what you have after you have been running and it is what you are because you run.

Ruth

I recently looked back at something I wrote when I was pregnant and pounding out the first draft of this book.

I was consumed with jealousy watching Olly go about his business this morning having kicked off his day with a run. I want to feel what he is feeling. I want a piece of that endorphin rush. I have to settle for a fast walk each day and I can tell you it is not the same. But, my body is being put to a different use for these coming months and I am determined to enjoy it. But, it got me thinking: how will I be able to fit in a run when the twins arrive? This will no doubt be a logistical nightmare, but I simply must find a way. Because I know that the hour I spend pounding Hampstead Heath will be the best hour I can invest in motherhood. It will give me those endorphins I'm desperate for, it will make the more dreary tasks of mothering more tolerable, and it will help me to snatch my sleep wherever I can get it. It will make the whole job that little bit easier to manage and give me energy and patience. And perhaps most importantly, it will help me to enjoy the babies and keep smiling. That's my theory anyway.

Ha – if only! The twins are now nine months old and the truth is that motivation meltdown struck me in a big way after they were born. I'd stopped running for short periods before: a few weeks, a few months even, but nothing like this. This was what I call TOTAL GLOBAL MELTDOWN. My body felt shattered by childbirth. Instead of feeling energised and empowered by the process, I lost all faith in my body. I was afraid of it all the time, afraid it would fail me. My bones seemed somehow to have moved into different positions and nothing seemed to work properly. There was no way I could run again. I decided instantly that my previous life was over and that I would never have the time or energy to run again. It took every ounce of physical strength I had just to stumble from one day to the next trying to manage with twins. I honestly thought I might die of tiredness. Running was out of the question.

But I kept getting these gently nudging emails from my agent about the book, which I had sent her just before the arrival of the twins, and I somehow managed to get through the early stages of preparing the book to go out to publishers. I wasn't running, but I was still thinking about running. I couldn't escape it. I tried to go on a run at Christmas time, but it was a disaster and served to confirm all my worst suspicions about my weak and ailing body. (Silly, on reflection, to run so soon and in such harsh conditions, too gritty altogether ... even for The Grit Doctor.) And then in the New Year my agent told me we had a publishing deal on the table. I was stunned and flabbergasted and felt a bit of a fraud. I hadn't run in eighteen months. I told myself it didn't matter because I had already written the book ... back when I was a different woman. But the deal came with a request for another 20,000 words. I found that I had nothing to say. Nothing funny or inspiring or real. I couldn't motivate myself to write at all, let alone write anything good, unless I started running again. And I just couldn't get myself back into it.

It struck me that this place – the place of TOTAL GLOBAL MELTDOWN – is actually the place where lots of people are at the very beginning. A place of no exercise and general apathy. I realised for the first time how very difficult it is to get started. Because after an eighteen-month gap, which included childbirth, my body had retained no running memory, no physical or emotional attachment to the exercise. I even stopped believing that it could be as good as all the things I had written about it. I had got used to a new way of being – one of resignation; that it was OK (and of course it is OK) to collapse on the sofa with a glass of wine after the twins were down for the night and ask Olly to order a takeaway. That it didn't really matter eating all that junk. I had stopped caring about my body even though it wasn't getting fat because the twins were burning up everything I had and then some, day after day, week after week, month after month. The bigger they got, the heavier they got and the more calories I burnt, so the more cake and junk I could eat. But I looked awful and I had no energy at all. I would collapse into bed at 9 p.m. each night and sleep fitfully until one of the babies woke me. But I was so used to this new way of being. I thought, I'm a mum now and this is how it is going to be. No time for anything except the babies and definitely no time to care about my body.

Two significant things happened, which I guess you could call catalysts:

Catalyst 1, Illness

The twins caught a bug. I caught it off them and I was completely poleaxed by it. Crawling around the house, cleaning up vomit and diarrhoea while unable to keep anything down myself, I was weak as a kitten. All I could do was cry. No sooner had I recovered from the bug when I came down with an awful cough which required antibiotics and took over a month to shift. Olly got the cough too, and needed two courses of antibiotics, inhalers, scans and all sorts to get right. I remembered that I never ever used to get ill when I was running. Somehow, running boosts your immune system and seems to guard against catching infections, colds and the like. Olly and I agreed that looking after the twins was impossible unless we were operating at 100%. We both knew that we needed to start running again, so that in turn we would start looking after our bodies better and caring more about what we were putting into them. Plus, deadlines were fast approaching for submitting the extra text for the book and my word count was a piddling few hundred. It was fear, really – for my health and of letting people down, of not getting the job done – that got me to stumble outside one spring evening after putting the twins down to bed, Olly just home from work. There was a part of me that was desperate to reclaim something of my former self, some of my old spark, to impress my husband who had been living with a shadow of the woman he had only recently fallen in love with. I walked to Highgate Wood (about ten minutes – the perfect warm up) went through the gates and started up the gentlest of trots ...

Catalyst 2, Injury

So Catalyst 1 was enough to get me into my trainers and out the front door. I had a slight twinge in my right knee, but fifteen minutes into the run it had disappeared. I ran slowly and deliberately and can honestly say at no point did I enjoy the run. It was brutal using those muscles again after so long and a gargantuan effort not to stop every five minutes. At no time did I enter any 'zone' other than the 'Go home NOW and STOP' zone. I was just praying I would complete what I had set out to do – a one-hour run around Highgate Wood. I did. My legs were like lead, and I thought with a start how out of touch with my body I had become. But I felt chuffed to bits with myself for having completed what I set out to do that day. Getting out the door once the twins were down, avoiding the fridge and the glass of vino, but using the thought of treating myself later to spur me on.

But no sooner had I set foot inside the house again, the magic started. I floated into the kitchen and straight over to the sink. I just wanted water. Gallons of it straight from the tap. It tasted like nectar. I immediately sat down at my computer and started writing. The words came easily and fluently and before I looked up I had written a thousand words. This is it. It's working. This is the magic that has been missing from my life. I felt energised. I felt happy. I felt knackered. I fell into bed that night and slept like a log for the first time since the last time I went running. I didn't wake to the tiny noises of the babies, not until the morning – 7.30 a.m., in fact, after about ten hours' sleep. It was the longest sleep I'd had since I was about four months pregnant.

I turned to get out of bed and that's when it happened. My right knee was agony. I looked at it, a swollen mass of flesh

*all tender and sore. Bugger. I was planning to go running
again that evening, write another thousand words etc. –
you get the picture. I had been scuppered at the first
hurdle. Lifting the babies and carrying them upstairs was
very difficult with the Elephant Man living inside your
knee, let me tell you. And I felt so depressed about it. And
anxious. Would I be able to write without running? Well, I
simply had to. And strangely, I was even more inspired by
the fact that I couldn't run. It had the same effect as the
pregnancy. Not allowed to run, rather than choosing not to.
Somehow, I turned the negative into a positive.*

ROPE IN A MATE

Now, I know that earlier I said that 'a problem shared is a
problem doubled'. Well, when you're a box-fresh runner,
starting out on Step 1 of The Grit Doctor's programme, that's
certainly true. But if you are a tired and jaded former runner
suffering from severe motivation meltdown, it can be really
useful to call on the support of your partner or a friend. Get
them to be your back-up Grit Doctor. It should be someone
whose respect you have earned and who you would be mor-
tified to let down. Tell this person that you intend to run and,
if necessary, get them to force you out of the door. Brief
them beforehand that you have no motivation, that you

know you will try everything in the book to get out of it and that it is their job to ensure that you get outside in your trainers and do not return for at least an hour. One of my excuses was that I couldn't find my trainers! Olly found them and put my feet into them and practically laced them up. If, after all that, I had failed to complete my run, the shame would have been too much to bear.

ALWAYS LIE ... TO YOURSELF

Lying can be a very useful motivating tool when cunningly deployed. I have been getting myself to go on runs lately by telling myself that I will go for a fast walk and run for just ten minutes and then come home. This gets me out of the door when I simply cannot face going for a run and my motivation is at an all-time low. It is brilliantly effective at getting you into your trainers and outside – which is always 90% of the battle – forcing you to take those first steps and get through that first awful ten minutes of *every* run. Because by the time you have done what you set out to do you will almost certainly want to go further. If motivation is still low after ten minutes, tell yourself another lie – just another five minutes and then home – and keep increasing the run by small increments if you are still struggling. Before you know it you have been running for an hour.

Ruth

After I'd signed my book deal, I went into my new publishers' offices to introduce them to The Grit Doctor and give a little talk about the book. I was terrified at the prospect of speaking to a room full of strangers, which made me feel particularly pathetic given that I am supposed to be a criminal barrister used to speaking in court. But presenting to a room full of strangers (interactive strangers!) is a very different animal to giving a speech to a stony-faced jury (who can't answer back) while wearing your wig, gown and glasses. I spoke to Olly about it the night before and asked his advice about how to get over the nerves. Other than the obvious 'go for a run' advice, he suggested owning up to how nervous I was.

I did just that and ended up talking about how running is a great metaphor for life and its challenges. I told them that I was going to approach the talk as I would a run. By doing it even though every part of my body and mind was telling me not to; by expecting the first ten minutes to be hellish and awful and then hoping to warm up a bit thereafter. I was also expecting there to be the odd twinge (and possibly some real pain) during the talk, but I hoped that at the end of it I would feel really chuffed with myself. That's what I said and it is exactly what happened. It turned out that many of the women in the room were interested in running and we had a really inspiring chat. One of the best areas of discussion was about getting yourself going. How do you turn on that switch to get yourself motivated? Isn't that the million dollar question, I thought aloud.

I pondered this question for some time after leaving the offices. How to flick the switch? And I came to the very gritty conclusion that there simply is no switch. Hoping for a switch to be turned on, the lights suddenly to go up and – abracadabra! – there you are, all bright-eyed, bushy-tailed and raring to go is just like hoping for a pill to make you thin or a knight in shining armour to make you happy. There is nothing you can take or 'turn on' to make you take those first steps outside. There is only you and your inner bitch. You have to harness something within you and make yourself go.

12

POST-BABY RUNNING ...
AND WHY RUNNING IS
BETTER THAN THERAPY

Running *tones your internal bullshit-o-meter ...*

Once you have got off your arse and completed the circuit that you thought you never could when you started out, you will realise that you can apply just the same gritty approach to everything else in your life that you resist. Think how long you fought against exercise and healthy eating. Consider the other stuff you may be resisting: moving job, dealing with relationship issues, having a clear-out, for example. Through the practice of running, you will become less tolerant of the nonsense that stops you from facing up to difficult stuff, and deal with it instead. It's probably due to a combination of the physiological 'happy' effect and a shift in attitude. But whatever the reason, running makes you tolerate less of your own bullshit, let alone other people's. And that is a very good thing.

My own motivation meltdown was entirely pregnancy-and baby-related, so I thought I should write a bit about my own experiences of the effect of pregnancy and childbirth on my runner's body and how I am dealing with it. Because I am still dealing with it. But I hope some of the advice here will be applicable to other runners who have been derailed for other reasons – perhaps a serious injury or illness.

The number one rule is this: do not go for a run too soon after childbirth – especially if you have had a C-section. I realise this should be obvious, but in my opinion the six-week no-exercise rule should be extended considerably when it comes to running. And this advice obviously applies to *any* serious operation. Not only should you be resting whenever you get the chance (as with a newborn you will be getting a total of three minutes' sleep a night) but your body has been through the equivalent of a car crash and needs time to repair itself. It needs rest to heal: the bones which shifted and the muscles that softened and relaxed in preparation for childbirth need time to adjust and strengthen again.

I was honestly afraid that everything might fall out – I felt very tender and protective of my womb area and nether regions. The hormone Relaxin softens all the muscles of the pelvic floor to allow your body to endure childbirth and your womb obviously has to deflate thereafter so that area feels very strange, entirely foreign in fact, for some time after delivery. Don't underestimate how fragile and tender you may feel for a while down there. Jumping up and down too soon (like I did) may put you off for good (as it nearly did to me).

Before you start any running at all, make sure you have been doing a lot of walking – ideally pushing your buggy, which is a great workout in itself and will slowly build up your fitness for that first run. And it's not just fitness that you need to build up. It's confidence. That was a real problem for me after having the twins. After a very traumatic birth, I was left feeling that my body was not up to any exercise and certainly not up to running.

FIRST-TIMERS

For the first-time runner who is also a first-time mum, you can just follow the programme in chapter 3, taking along your buggy to establish the circuit if you wish. But DON'T RUN WITH THE BUGGY until you are a confident runner. Once you have an established running routine and feel the need to challenge yourself, feel free to join the pushy mothers brigade and kill two birds with one stone: get your baby outside for some fresh air and give yourself a fantastic workout. Be sure to use an appropriate buggy, i.e. one that is designed to allow you to run and push. NOT YOU,

MOTHERS OF MULTIPLES. It is not safe to run with your double buggy, nor remotely sane, and you absolutely need to get away from those babies for your run. The Grit Doctor's orders.

It is perfectly safe to run while breastfeeding (obviously not actually *during* a breastfeed) but you will need to take extra care with hydration and nutrition. Simply put, eat more and drink more water. The right bra is crucial and, of course, nursing pads to deal with leakage.

I would actually suggest waiting until your baby is sleeping through the night before you start running. Maybe I am less gritty than I thought, but I tried to run three months in and was so knackered afterwards that I found the nightshift almost impossible. Perhaps if I'd carried on it would have been different, but that one run, too soon, put me off trying again for another three months.

OLD-TIMERS

If you ran before your pregnancy, you should expect to feel different after it so don't expect to be able to go at it hammer and tongs like you did before. Not straight away, that is. However, you are the best judge of your limits. Go for a short, slow run and take your temperature – metaphorically speaking – once you have been given the all-clear by your

GP. If you are a Paula Radcliffe type, clearly you will be able to run a marathon and win it very soon thereafter. Having a baby is no reason or excuse to think you are not up to it any more. You absolutely are, and may well enjoy the happiest, sexiest time of your life post-babies. Not only that, you may end up with an even better body! And do take full advantage of that feeling that you can conquer the world because you survived giving birth to fuel your running addiction and lust for life. You can do anything and you will transform that desire into action through a committed running practice. Just be prepared for your body to feel a bit different now.

THE GRIT DOCTOR SAYS:

You may be lacking in iron and calcium post-childbirth so take a supplement if necessary. It will become another thing that you are doing for yourself – taking care of your body, which is a very positive thing indeed.

POSTNATAL DEPRESSION

For the love of God, look after yourself and do what your real doctor tells you, not The Grit Doctor! I was really down for a long time after the twins were born. The sleep deprivation was probably the main cause, but I now realise that the lack of exercise was also a major factor. The twins were born in late September so those early months were pretty grim, night feeds in the dark and early morning starts in the dark – hideous. My motivation and confidence were at an all-time low. Medication for post-natal depression combined with regular running was hugely healing for me and certainly helped lift and regulate my moods. Notwithstanding this, if you have been diagnosed with postnatal depression (no self-diagnosis please) do ask your GP if you can start the Six-Step Programme. My feeling is that it would be wholeheartedly endorsed as very good therapy indeed.

HOW TO GET YOURSELF OUT THERE AGAIN

- I get into my running clothes and trainers during the afternoon when the twins are having a nap so I am mentally prepared that after their day is ended, I am out of the door.

- I text Olly during the afternoon and tell him I want to go for a run the minute he gets home and to make me go if I try and wriggle out of it. He is my back-up Grit Doctor.

- I plan something totally delicious and massive for dinner as a reward and get Olly involved in preparing it while I am out running and fantasise about it during the run.

- I lie to myself. As mentioned above, an hour's run in ten-minute increments is a cunning trick which gets me out of the door in the first place and then all the way around my route.

- Throughout the day I want to go running and during the run itself I repeat this mantra, stolen from a great friend who supplied a case study for the book: *Every time you run, you win. Even a bad run is a win. Small win after small win. Day after day. WHEN YOU RUN, RUTH, YOU WIN.* It gives me shivers up and down my spine and propels me forward. Use it or find one of your own: a pithy line that gets you going and fires you up. 'RUN FAT BITCH RUN' is always a good one to fall back on.

And think of all the benefits you'll get from just LEAVING THE HOUSE and stretching your body and mind.

- Freedom from all your responsibilities. It is temporary (unless you keep on running ... but I'm not for one moment suggesting that, however tempting it might sometimes seem!) but it feels amazing that for an hour you can be completely on your own again.

- Rediscovery of yourself as a woman rather than just as a wife and mother.

- Re-sculpting all of the muscles and body tone lost since childbirth.

- Creative thinking.

- A sense of incredible peace.

- Exploring the beauty of nature and your local community without the buggy. Taking in all the nooks and crannies that it prevents you from getting to.

- Unbeatable fat-burning exercise and cardio workout.

- A phenomenal night's sleep during which you won't wake to every tiny noise that the baby makes.

- Renewed confidence and motivation as a mother.

- Increased love and patience for your baby and partner.

- Energy to do all of your chores and to enjoy looking after the baby.

- Enhanced sexual drive with the increased energy and appetite for life!

- Determination to go running again and keep trying to improve in all areas.

That hour is YOU time. You won't be able to fill this hour with mothering or wife-ing (which you *will do* if you stay indoors). It's all about *you* for an hour – for once! For your thoughts. For your body. For your mind. And it works. It really works. You'll come back refreshed and happy. Feeling more loving towards your partner and seeing your baby again for the miracle he/she is. And you will start to take care of yourself again – your body and mental well-being so taken over by the baby's needs. It is truly awesome. But The Grit Doctor accepts it requires an awesome amount of effort, too.

RUNNING FOR YOUR LIFE

Running can help you cope with all sorts of struggles. A great friend of mine, who I knew had taken up running in the last few years, wrote a very moving account of how running helped her during a tremendously difficult time.

```
To: The Grit Doctor

From: A friend

Re: My Affair With Running
```

The secret I kept hidden was that I
started running as an escape. The escape
was psychological as well as physical: not
from the insistent demands of a baby and
toddler as everyone assumed, not
particularly as an escape from the effects
on my body of two pregnancies and too much
consumption, but as an escape from the
crushing weight of domestic abuse.

Always conscious of my size (often
described as 'robust'), my figure was a
battleground and I was rarely the victor.
A moment of enlightenment came when, with
the children in the bike trailer, I almost
failed to go half a mile, halted by the
mildest incline which would not even merit
the word 'hill'. At the same time, my
marriage was coming back into focus after
the distractions of babies, a move and a
new job. In reality, the patterns of abuse
had always been there, subtly in the
background. The immediate pressures of
working parenthood were just increasing
the difficulties, and my determination to

be the best mother I could, and work to the best of my abilities, meant that my husband's sense of displacement was coupled with anger and aggression. Aggression that ranged from passive to most certainly active. I was frequently told I was fat and unattractive and sex became an area of increasingly hostile discontent. So, a part of the plan to 'sort out' the marriage was to remedy the 'fat' side of things and I hoped that that, along with a barrage of other strategies, would hopefully change my husband's behaviour.

So I started running, only because it was the most exercise I could do in the shortest time away from the children and the house. The smallest circuit was one-and-a-half miles and a stitch would inevitably come within the first half mile. Then the stitch would come later, then the circuit was stitch free. Next came a longer route — three miles with a hill — then six miles became the staple circuit, and so it built up. With longer runs, I escaped more and felt mentally free. But with longer runs, the anger increased and I was faced with the choice of a run plus anger, a longer run plus more anger or no run, and discontentment and still anger from my husband.

At one point, my husband said it was like I was having an affair. Only the affair was with running. The evidence? He fixed me with a steely stare, felt under the bed and brandished his evidence. *Running World* magazine.

The more I ran, the more anger and abuse I was escaping from. The crunch came when I began a weekly half-marathon circuit. Two hours, I was told, was not acceptable. Nine hours of cricket was, apparently, perfectly fine.

I sought counselling but then I was banned from going by my husband. The counsellor had picked up on the abuse instantly and advised me to get out of the marriage for the safety of the children. The situation would inevitably spiral down, she said.

Thinking I could change the situation, and with some resentment, I decreased my running and tried another battery of marriage saving strategies. But the desire to run, to escape, remained. As predicted, things spiralled: the anger exploded, the abuse worsened. Running became my only coping mechanism, my natural Prozac, and I came to rely completely on its power of escape and its effects psychologically and physiologically.

My now ex-husband finally left and once the locks were changed, the feeling of safety seeped back into my life — a feeling so underappreciated in my earlier life and a feeling I still revel in. It's a feeling similar to the high of running: that you are free, that you are uninhibited and you could keep running forever.

I recently met up with this friend. She is still going through a fairly messy divorce but is coping brilliantly, and is using running to help keep her sane.

HOW RUNNING CAN CURE HEARTACHE

Nothing cures a broken heart like a good run. I ran my way through the pain after being dumped one Christmas Eve and came out the other side in springtime looking and feeling great. A run will inevitably make you feel less sad and less deranged (because of the happy hormones). Equally, in running you are caring for your body in a way that heartbreak might otherwise prevent you from doing. Instead of starving and wallowing and drinking yourself into an early grave, by running you are cherishing your body and bruised heart. In keeping fit and looking good you will give your self-confidence a much-needed boost. My sister's best friend Polly recently told me that running has cured her heartbreak – well, almost.

To: The Grit Doctor

From: Polly

Re: One Foot in Front of the Other

I can't sleep, I don't feel hungry, I
can't set my mind to anything for more
than a few minutes, my whole body hurts
and I feel sick. And then I run. Running
is the best antidote to heartbreak I've
ever known.

When I run I can focus my mind in the
most rational way; I don't over-think and
as I focus on putting one foot in front
of the other, I can order my feelings
about him and the panic subsides.
Equally, I can let all thoughts of him
fall out of my mind, empty my head and
think of nothing at all except the sound
of my breathing and footfall and snippets
of strangers' conversations.

Running is the purest way I have found to deal with the seemingly endless ache. The pain doesn't go away completely but it is far more bearable and I am, at least, starving and physically exhausted rather than numb when I run every day. I feel so lively when I've done my few miles and I look forward to the next day when I can get the rush again — it's the healthiest addiction I've ever had. And I hope that if and when I ever see him again, I will look incredible.

And she does — look incredible that is.

13

WHEN THE ADDICTION
TAKES HOLD ...

Running teaches you to enjoy your own company ...
   This is something that my husband pointed out to me
recently, that he has really started to relish that time on
his own (time away from The Grit Doctor perhaps?).
Some of you may already be lovers of your own
company – I certainly am – in which case there is nothing
better than getting to indulge that side of your
personality, whenever you feel the urge, by going off for a
run. This can be especially handy if you are in a situation
with loads of people and need to escape. No one is
going to criticise you for going off for a run (they might if
you snuck off to the pub without inviting anyone). I'm
thinking Christmas at home, surrounded by family and
friends when you're frankly sick to death of the lot of
them. Go for a run, and not only will that hour be pure
heaven, it will give you the strength and patience to deal
with the rest of your time at home. Better still, you may
actually relax and enjoy it.

SHARE THE LOVE, BUT BEWARE THE *OVER*SHARE

For God's sake, don't talk about running all the time. I know I am, but I am writing a book to help you. You wouldn't, however, catch me talking about this stuff at a dinner party. Food and exercise talk is very low-grade chat. Much more interesting and inspiring to just BE the amazing person you have become through running: contented, peaceful, energised and invigorating company. Be sure to try and encourage and motivate others but not by lecturing. Buy this book for your mate instead and spread the word that way. Wait until someone notices that you look a whole lot better – thinner and happier – and only then casually mention what you are doing:

'Thanks. Actually, I've taken up running.'

'Wow, how did you get started?'

'Well, it was surprisingly easy. I read this amazing book and just got on with it really.'

And leave it at that. Don't ram it down people's necks. Let them ask for help first. There are three obvious exceptions to the 'don't talk about it' rule. Obviously, it's a good idea to spill the beans over a deep and meaningful catch-up with your best mate. The second exception is before, during and after a race with fellow competitors. The third is if you ever find yourself at a dinner party made up entirely of fanatical runners. Go for it. Unleash the beast. Who knows where it might lead . . .

If you're a keen runner living with a bona fide coach potato, the temptation to evangelise about the benefits of running can be too much to bear. I definitely *over*shared my running enthusiasm when Olly and I first met and totally put him off. But eventually I figured out that subtle demonstrations of the benefits of running were far more effective than lecturing him and he is now, as we have seen, transforming into a lean, mean, running machine. Quality 'sharing', delivered in the right way, at the right time, is nothing short of an artform – the deployment of which requires great skill and ingenuity. Get it wrong and you lose your audience. Get it right, however, and you can change lives. What follows is what I recommend if you too share your life with a long-term running-phobe.

- *Do not* manically bang on about the benefits of running. It will do nothing to convert the non-believer. Olly thought it was very weird, cult-like and boring to hear any running chat whatsoever and made that clear very early on in our relationship.

- **Do** exploit opportunities to stand next to him naked in the mirror (remember Delusions of *Thinneur* are doubly true when you are in denial *and* are overweight). Resist the urge to make comments or gasp in dismay, but do stand in such a way that accentuates as much as possible the differences between you.

- **Do** continue running and slyly *demonstrate*, not advocate, in as many ways as you can the many post-run benefits. For example: improved mood; sleeping like a log; eating like a horse; having an insatiable sexual appetite.

- **Do** take advantage of any opportunity to drink gallons of water in front of him while pretending to enjoy it and making appropriate noises of appreciation.

- **Do** lead by example on the food front. Always make healthy food choices in his company and eat to your heart's content. It will no doubt irritate and confuse him enormously that you seem to eat as much, if not more, than he does, yet remain super-toned. Gently explain that you go running every day which burns off a lot of fuel and that's why you can eat so much and that it's great isn't it!

- **Do not** forget his male pride. Remember he is a man. Don't emphasise your infinite superiority in such a way as to totally humiliate him – this is likely to put him off for good (off running and you).

- **Do** encourage him *when he deserves it* and give appropriate honest compliments. When he tells you what a beautiful, toned, slim, fit body you have, do not respond by telling him the same thing about himself. He doesn't. Instead say, 'You could too, darling, it's just because I run, it keeps me in such good shape.'

- **Do** set the best possible example in sticking to your running routine and demonstrating your self-discipline in other areas of your life. When asked, always acknowledge that running is the reason why. Before long, and with a bit of luck, your other half will be so inspired by you, that he will join the club. If not out of inspiration, then competition may win the day, because no one likes to be outshone by their other halves. In the end he will want a piece of the action.

ADVANCED RUNNING

THE GRIT DOCTOR SAYS:

The Grit Doctor is all for pushing yourself further, stepping outside of your comfort zone and becoming the best version of yourself.

Some of you will get obsessed with running and The Grit Doctor is keen that you take advantage of this zeal.

All of you who have completed the Six-Step Programme and are able to run for forty-five minutes without stopping, at least three times a week, are more than ready to enter a 5 km race. DO IT. Racing is amazing and so motivating. There will be numerous local 5 km's you can enter (see Appendix 2, or ask at your local running shop). Now is a great time to rope in a mate – maybe someone you know who is a runner but who doesn't yet know you are? Invite them to enter a 5 km race with you. Just stick to what you are doing, running regularly, and that is all the training you need to do. Unless, of course, you plan on winning the race, in which case work through the training programme which follows and run like the wind on race day!

INCREASING DISTANCES

Now that you are so much fitter and able to complete your circuit easily (and crucially, in less time) you can squeeze in some extra mileage. You should be able to go from 3–4 miles to 4–5 miles quite effortlessly and enjoy the extra high you will get from your regular run. Don't attempt to progress from a 4-mile to an 8-mile run overnight. Use the same strategies for increasing distance you employed during the Six-Step Programme – slow and steady all the way.

Fitting in a long run over the weekend is a great way to

increase your fitness and stamina. An 8-miler will really satisfy your running lust and take you to a whole new world of satisfaction.

RUN OFF-PISTE

Go somewhere completely different. Plan a new run beforehand. Take in more cross-country. You don't need to follow anything other than your animal instinct for increased fitness and challenges. Go for it. But don't get complacent. Motivation meltdown will still hit you. YES. IT. WILL. Sometimes the higher you've climbed the further you have to fall. So never take it for granted. Remember the importance of routine in your daily running regime. By all means go crazy once in a while, or when you're visiting somewhere new, but try to keep to your established route on your regular runs.

To: The Grit Doctor

From: Olly

Re: Striking Out

Once I'd cracked my original circuit, it gave me the confidence to start striking out on different routes and really explore the countryside around the village. I ran down every road or pathway that I could find, just to see where it would take me. Along the way I'd peer into people's houses, speculate wildly on their occupations and relationships, and generally have a good nose around.

I found a great run which took me past a grand-looking chateau and up through some woods to some ruins on the outskirts of town, and another which took me past an abandoned Renault parked in a ditch, a field full of horses and a converted chapel. Such was my sudden desire to push myself that I even got Ruth to take me to the local football pitch to do interval training with me. In other words, she stood in the middle of the field while I ran round the edge and every so often shouted 'SPRINT!' at me. I actually

> volunteered for it. I actually enjoyed it.
> Although not, I suspect, quite as much as
> Ruth did.

CONCRETE ADVICE

The reason that running on concrete *seems* so much easier is because it is, in fact, much easier. You bounce straight off it almost as soon as your feet touch the ground. To the novice this can be seductive, but for all the wrong reasons. You will be able to go for longer and won't feel so knackered so quickly, which is why it is very important indeed not to get fooled by concrete in the early stages of your running career and start as you mean to go on, on the softer surfaces. Grass is the best. Trails and dirt tracks a close second. Yes, it feels difficult. Yes, it is hard. Hard is the new black remember? (Repeat this to yourself as you get stuck in the mud.) One day you may be able to run barefoot on sand. Now THAT is something for the seasoned sado-masochist. The ache in those calves and butt is like nothing you have ever known.

To: The Grit Doctor

From: Father Henry Wansbrough

Re: Extreme Running

I used to coach rugby and athletics at the monastery attached to the school where I taught, and after athletics in the summer we would often run over to the lake on the edge of the school grounds as a wind-down and have a swim. On other days I would go for a run by myself, so I got into the habit. That is when I do a lot of my thinking, preparing lectures or classes. It is lovely countryside with great views and I find the solitude and tranquillity very healing.

There are some woods nearby with a thousand different paths — I can still get lost there after running in them for fifty years and more. That adds an element of excitement. When I go to lecture or teach in other monasteries it is very relaxing to get out and away from everything and explore the countryside — after a few days I often find I know it better than the inhabitants themselves, though I only go about 5-8 miles. Again there is a certain amount of adventure. In Kenya I was almost attacked by a buffalo. In Zimbabwe I ran up the Zambezi, got hot and dived in for a swim, quite unaware that it was full of crocodiles. In the USA I went running in the morning on a broad empty road and then as the traffic built up discovered that it was an interstate highway.

I suppose the most important thing which starts me up again is the need for solitude and simply the enjoyment of the grass, the wild flowers and the trees. It is said that there are puma in those woods too ...

Father Wansbrough, who used to teach my brothers, is over eighty years old and still runs most days.

The Grit Doctor wants you to win. The great thing about running is that just by setting out on a run, every time you put one foot in front of the other you win. And entering a race is a big win. In committing to a race and training programme you have already won. After that, it's up to you to decide what constitutes a win. Set yourself a time, try and outdo a friend, try and beat the person running just a bit in front of you at the end. How many people you overtake. That sort of thing. All are wins. *Every time you put one foot in front of the other you win – that is the beauty of running.*

Ruth

When I told my mother that I was running the London Marathon, she got herself into a bit of a tizz about it, which I thought was weird. She didn't want to come to London to watch me run – she said she was too nervous and it was only the night before the marathon that I discovered why. She called me up and burst out,

> *'Darling, promise me one thing?'*
> *'What, Mum?'*
> *'That you won't try and win it.'*

Unbelievable. My mother had visions of me up in the front trying to overtake Paula Radcliffe. I wish. I was bemused and very flattered. Such is my competitive streak that my mother could not envisage me entering a race and not trying to win it. She then complained bitterly afterwards that she hadn't seen me on the TV ... clearly she had been looking in all the wrong places, i.e. a few paces behind Paula.

OPTIONAL EXTRAS FOR ADDED GRIT FACTOR

The Grit Doctor does not want you to get sidetracked by other exercises in the early stages of your running programme (because of the inevitable time-wasting involved), but once you've mastered the running and are trying to push yourself, and if you are tough enough, then doing some sit-ups, press-ups and pull-ups at the end of your run is fantastic. Yes, just lie down on a patch of grass and get on with it. This will help strengthen and improve core muscle groups which ultimately will improve your running. You will also look hard as nails and cool as ...

FOOD AND DRINK

If you're training more, eat more – if you fancy it. You can, because you will be burning it off. Drink more water. And take water on your long run. Isotonic drinks are unnecessary for training at this level and will only add a huge number of wasted calories to your daily intake – calories which would be better spent on a massive meal and a few celebratory drinks afterwards.

The real test of your running mettle is entering a race. A *real* race. A 5 km should be easy as pie for you now, so push yourself further by entering a 10 km, with the ultimate goal of one day, maybe, entering a marathon. With race training, for a 10 km as much as a marathon, it's all about gradually increasing distance and building up stamina using interval and hill training. These techniques are covered in depth in Part 4's Marathon Plan, as well as the 10 km training plan which follows.

14

THE GRIT DOCTOR'S 10 KM TRAINING PLAN

Running boosts your confidence . . .

   This was a benefit I certainly had not anticipated when I took up running, but it is very real. And it doesn't just come from the better body you get and which you will be keen to show off. You will start to feel confident in all other areas of your life – at work and on dates for example. In fact, confidence is one of the best benefits and surprising side effects of running. Good self-esteem and confidence are the bedrocks of happiness and success after all (they also enable you to make better friends with your inner bitch). With confidence, your life opens up and the possibilities are endless. Sounds unbelievably cheesy, I know. But it's true.

THE GRIT DOCTOR RECOMMENDS:

Use your working week as a template to train for the 10 km – with your serious training taking place on weekdays. There is one very important exception: do not make Monday the worst day. (Mondageddon is not the way to start any week, The Grit Doctor always eases herself into a Monday.) Take Friday as your rest day, Saturday as your long run day and Sunday for your easy run, that way you feel as though you are getting a bit of a weekend. Don't feel you have to follow this slavishly, remember to use your initiative and adapt schedules to suit yourself. Just be sure to take a rest day, but don't overdo it – the resting that is. And always keep in tune with that body of yours – listen to it carefully and stick to the grass and trails as much as you can.

---

10 km is equivalent to 6.2 miles, and, unless you are super-woman, this is further than you have been running thus far during your forty-five-minute, thrice-weekly jog. You could run it without training if you just continued to run as you are, but in order to enjoy it and stretch yourself, I recommend stepping up your regime. Below is a rough guide to what I did when training to run in a 10 km a few years back.

THE GRIT DOCTOR SAYS:

It is not a train crash if you miss a session, or swap sessions, or change your rest days – the keys to success at 10 km are some interval training to improve your stamina and speed and getting a longer run in each week to increase your distances. Try to incorporate some hill running into your longer weekend run if possible as this is a fantastic way to improve your powers of endurance.

WEEK 1

Monday

If possible, do some exercise today other than running: cross training, swimming or a sexathon are perfect. If this is impossible because you burnt your gym membership (The Grit Doctor applauds you for this) or do not have a willing partner, don't worry. Other types of exercise are in no way crucial to your success at 10 km. Go on a very short run or a long walk and/or have a good rest. Mondays are essentially Fundays to be spent as you so wish. The grit begins tomorrow.

Tuesday

As with all running, interval training requires you to warm up first, so do your usual brisk walk to get your muscles relaxed. Run slowly for the first 400m then speed up for as long as you can manage (if you count to 100 in your head while sprinting and can manage that, great. If you can go for longer even better). Then jog very slowly again for roughly 400m then quickly for as long as you can manage – up to 400m ideally. Don't worry if you can barely make it to 50m the first few times. You will improve. Keep it up for 30 minutes.

THE GRIT DOCTOR SAYS:

For the first timer, interval training makes the new black look even blacker. But you are going to learn to LOVE it.

Wednesday

Forty to forty-five minutes of easy running. By that I mean your usual forty-five-minute run.

Thursday

Interval training again as per Tuesday.

Friday

Rest, relax and enjoy yourself.

Saturday

Longer run for an hour (about 5 miles) at your normal pace.

Sunday

Forty to forty-five minutes of easy running.

A GRIT DOCTOR REMINDER:

Do not ignore your rest days. Your muscles repair and restore themselves during rest periods, enabling you to improve and stretch them thereafter.

WEEK 2

Monday As per Week 1

Tuesday As per Week 1, but try to extend your sprints and up the pace, even if it's only by a few metres

Wednesday As per Week 1

Thursday As per Week 1 Tuesday

Friday REST

Saturday Long run – 5.5 miles

Sunday As per Week 1

WEEK 3

Monday As per Week 1

Tuesday As per previous week, but up the ante on both pace and length of sprints where you can. Keep it up for 40 mins

Wednesday As per Week 1

Thursday As per Tuesday

Friday REST

Saturday Long run – 6 miles

Sunday As per Week 1

WEEK 4

Monday As per Week 1

Tuesday As per previous week, but extend overall length of run to include more intervals. 45 mins overall

Wednesday As per Week 1

Thursday As per Tuesday or take on a hill instead. Keep it up for 45 mins (not uphill for the entirety, please)

Friday REST

Saturday Long run – 7 miles

Sunday As per Week 1

THE GRIT DOCTOR SAYS:

Your interval training sessions are where your speed and endurance improve. They always feel uber gritty. This is entirely the point. So expect to dread them and never hope that they will be fun. *Grittify* them wherever possible by increasing sprinting distances and/or by speeding up the sprints. If you like to run against the clock or be very specific about distances, do set yourself targets, increasing them by small increments each week until week 7. Hill running is another excellent way to improve your fitness and speed and you can always swap one weekly interval training session with a hill run. It may seem like a welcome break a few weeks into your plan so do mix them into it. Your normal runs and even that longer weekend run are going to feel so easy by comparison!

WEEK 5

Monday REST

Tuesday As per previous week, but really nail those sprints as fast as you can manage

Wednesday As per Week 1

Thursday As per Tuesday or hill training if you prefer

Friday REST

Saturday Long run – 8 miles

Sunday As per Week 1

WEEK 6

Monday As per Week 1

Tuesday As per previous week, enjoying those sprints now?!

Wednesday As per Week 1

Thursday What hill?!

Friday REST

Saturday Long run – 8 miles

Sunday As per Week 1

WEEK 7

Monday REST

Tuesday As per previous week, 40 mins overall

Wednesday As per Week 1

Thursday Short, sharp fast sprints, 30 mins

Friday REST

Saturday Long run – 6 miles

Sunday As per Week 1

WEEK 8

Monday REST

Tuesday 45 mins easy running

Wednesday REST

Thursday 30 mins interval/hill run

Friday REST

Saturday RACE DAY. Best of luck and may the grit be with you

Sunday SLEEP, EAT AND DRINK A LOT (of water, too)!

PART 4

THE MARATHON PLAN

15

INTRODUCTION TO THE MARATHON PLAN

FIRST THINGS FIRST

I'm going to assume you've been nailing forty-five-minute runs three times a week, minimum, and have morphed into a runner of sorts. If not, why not? Do so now. You really need to master the basics before you attempt the marathon. If you have just finished a 10k, as I have, and are wanting to up the ante right away, as I am, signing up for a half-marathon is the perfect way to satisfy your race-hungry legs. DO IT NOW. There will be plenty within striking distance of your home and far enough in the future for you to be race-ready. I have never run one myself, having signed up for the London Marathon all those years ago without so much as a mile under my belt. Madness. So I have just signed up for the Bristol half-marathon, four months from now. And I'm feeling pumped about it. Remember though, the half-marathon is effectively double the furthest distance you have run so far. Treat it with respect. The training programme I have devised follows on naturally from my 10k programme and assumes you can run 10k *without stopping* relatively comfortably (I use 'comfortably' in The Grit Doctor sense of the word).★

THE GRIT DOCTOR SAYS:

If you have the undeniable, if slightly mad, urge to sign up for a full marathon right now, DO IT. Don't waste a second contemplating the pros and cons in your head.

Turn to the Applying for a Marathon chapter in the back of the book for information on how to apply for the London Marathon – the World Cup of 26-milers – and other marathons and half-marathons in the UK and overseas.

TRUE GRIT

★Other than the half-marathon training programme, the majority of references will be about the marathon. The full 26.2 miles. However, everything I say about the marathon applies to a 13-miler too – just be sensible about the carb loading if you are only doing a half and have no intention of going the full distance *pulls slightly disappointed face*.

The bottom line is this: the marathon is all about the runs; the runs you have to put in, day after day, week after week. The runs that will transform you into someone capable of going the whole distance. While it may be interesting and useful to research the subject, no amount of study is going to make that happen for you. So, read, research, fanny around in shops, surf the net, join a group – yes – but not at the expense of even a single extra mile of training.

THE GRIT DOCTOR SAYS:
Every mile that you bank now will pay dividends on race day. BEGIN NOW.

WHAT DOES THE GRIT DOCTOR HAVE TO OFFER ME?

This marathon plan is different from the rest in three ways. Firstly, **running a marathon is not really about *running* the marathon**. Yep, suck it up folks. Of course, the same doesn't apply to Paula Radcliffe, who is clearly in it to win it, but I'm not here to teach a granny to suck eggs. This might seem like a bit of a curve ball, but it will all become clear later. Secondly, one of the best things about entering, training for and running a marathon, BY MILES, is that you can

stuff your face with carbs on a daily basis and still look a million times hotter than any of your friends.* This book is really going to celebrate the carb in a big way. By way of whetting those appetites, let me tell you that one of the staple marathon-training foods I will be advocating is the PIE. *The pie will be your diet.* OK, not literally, but where the pie was a borderline 'Seven Deadly Sins' foodstuff in *RFBR* (on account of the pastry), when you're a marathon runner it becomes something you can devour guilt-free. Not possible! I hear you object. Pies are unhealthy and crap, surely? Not the pies you'll find here, just waiting to be brought to life in your kitchens – they're full of ideal foodstuffs to fuel your marathon training and delicious to boot. I will also show you how to recognise good carbs from bad and a fuss-free way of working out what to eat, and how much, so you don't get too bogged down thinking about food and can concentrate on the important stuff – the runs. The third and perhaps most crucial difference is **the tone**. As you know The Grit Doctor's tone is harsh – brutal, even – but also funny and *incredibly motivating*. And the marathon is all about motivation. So, through a combination of tough love and humour, the occasionally dry information on the page will be magically transformed into inspiration for your training programme.

---

*I'm afraid this does not apply if you are morbidly obese and have never run, yet entered a marathon for reasons best known to yourself. Step away from the pies. STEP AWAY FROM THE PIES. Concentrate on getting yourself moving and shedding those excess pounds.

WHAT IS GRIT AND WHY DO I NEED IT?

Dictionary definition of grit (other than the obvious granular, sandy one): **Firmness of character; indomitable spirit; pluck.**

The Grit Doctor is *loving* the word pluck. Those three qualities are what it means to be gritty – strong, unstoppable and brave. And to acquire and hone them requires shed-loads of discipline. It doesn't matter if you are weak-willed, fearful and the most lazy person on the planet, in training for a marathon you will become the very embodiment of those qualities. You cannot run a marathon without discipline, and the discipline of character you develop over your training schedule will ultimately translate into a discipline on race day, step by step, mile by mile.

THE GRIT DOCTOR SAYS:

Pluck is the new black.

Good, old-fashioned grit is what will make you push your-self, what will stop you bailing on your training sessions and make you stretch yourself during each run. On race day, it is what will drive you to achieve your goal. It is what will keep you putting one foot in front of another. Because that is what all this boils down to, from the moment you sign up until the moment you cross the finishing line: putting one foot in front of the other. Pretty straightforward, really. And yet, before you reach that finishing line, no matter how good your training was and no matter what sort of incredible physical shape you are in, you will still reach a place of tortuous mental derangement where every fibre of your being, every muscle, every sinew, every cell in your brain is screaming out at you to stop. In that moment it is the voice of The Grit Doctor and your Inner Bitch who will be there to propel you onwards.

THE GRIT DOCTOR SAYS:

OK, intros over. Go for a run, clear your head and ponder developing firmness of character, indomitable spirit and pluck: GET GRITTY.

Ruth

You already know that I ran two marathons many years ago. I think it's best I 'fess up to this one right from the start: I ran the London Marathon in four hours and forty minutes, or thereabouts, and New York the following year in around five-and-a-half hours. I think. (Hampered, if you recall, by my promise to remain at the side of my flatmate.) In both marathons I suffered from lack of training, in not leaving a long enough gap between entering the marathon and running it to complete a proper training programme.

THE GRIT DOCTOR SAYS:

There is nothing that can substitute for training. Not youth, not enthusiasm, not anything. No exceptions.

What got me to the end of both marathons without ever stopping was my Inner Bitch – The Grit Doctor – who never let me stop, not even for a second, not even when I had to jog backwards to keep my friend company nor when I hit The Wall at mile 22 of the London Marathon. So what I lacked in training, I made up for in grit. I reckon those times would have been a whole lot worse but for the ever-present shouty voice in my head that kept me going in the face of my body's screams to stop. I also reckon they could get a whole lot better with a more realistic and better organised training programme.

16

MOTIVATION – BECOME A GRIT MACHINE

It is a huge thing to commit to training for and running a marathon and in so doing you will experience an immediate shift in your attitude to your fitness, to training, to commitment. And we should all acknowledge what an achievement it is to take that leap and sign up. The courage it takes to say yes to such a challenge is enormous, and the action of doing just that may well give you a huge initial injection of motivation. Capitalise on this immediately by going for a run – a big one! The difficult thing with marathon running is sustaining that motivation throughout the training period, which may be six months or possibly anything up to a year. And that is where The Grit Doctor comes in.

KILLING OFF MOTIVATION

At marathon-level training, a complete shift in attitude to motivation is required in order to succeed. Motivation needs to become the icing on the cake, not the cake itself. By that I mean, when all our training is done and dusted, when we are at the end of our run, then – and only then – should we be calling upon our reserves of motivation to go an extra mile, to take on an extra hill, to squeeze in an extra session of strength training. At marathon-level training we should not be wasting time and expending energy – *ever* – on the question 'if . . . ?', but only on 'when?' and 'for how long?' and 'how fast?' will I run today? Obviously, this isn't easy to achieve and some days in training for the Bristol Half Marathon I am still totally stuck in the vicious motivation cycle: shall I, shan't I go for a run? So this is the ideal state that we should be aspiring to and working towards – a motivation-less state – because when it does work it is incredibly effective, and fitting in my runs becomes so much simpler and miles quicker! I don't ask myself whether I am motivated to eat or have a shower. As a result I do these things completely naturally, without pause or question.

THE GRIT DOCTOR SAYS:
Action destroys fear.

YOU HAVE ALREADY WON

Entering a marathon or a half-marathon is a huge win. 'Winning' never means being up there smashing world records with the Kenyans, unless you happen to be a Kenyan and/or a world-record contender, of course. A 'win' will mean something completely different for every person reading this.

Now just so we are clear, entering and completing the marathon at *any time* is a win. It is up to you to decide, within that, what constitutes a win *for you*. Once you have decided what that is, it is my job to help keep you on track. For some of you just walking the 26 miles will be a win, for others it might be wearing a fancy-dress costume and taking twelve hours to lug it around the course, while others *will* be expecting to be up there with the Kenyans (and possibly not wasting any time reading this book). Some of you will aim to raise £500 or £5000 for charity, others will race to stick two fingers up to a serious or even terminal illness. It doesn't matter what your win is *so long as you do win*. And win you will if you are able to cultivate your relationship with your Inner Bitch and harness that voice for strength and motivation.

LOSERS

Where there are winners there must also be losers. Don't be one of them. A 'lose' in the context of your marathon is simply failing to achieve your goal, whatever it was. So, if you decided a win for you would be completing the marathon in four hours and you completed it in 4.01, you have lost. You still did bloody well, but let us be clear – a win is a win is a win and you *only win* if you achieve what you set out to do. It helps to be strict about this because it will keep you focused and motivated during training. Declare early on what your win is going to be and then start training with it always at the forefront of your mind. You can always up the ante later on – for example, by changing your goal time from 1/2 hours to 4.15 – but I hope you will never lower your goal. So, thoughtful consideration ought to be given to your decision as to what constitutes your win, before making your declaration. Be realistic but be bold and brave too.

THE GRIT DOCTOR SAYS:

After careful consideration, declare your win to the world and keep your actions and choices consistent with it.

Ruth

I have just signed up for my first half-marathon. I have four months until race day and am able to run 10k in just shy of an hour. I want to run the half-marathon in under two hours. That would constitute a win for me. So now my training, my running, my very being, must begin to reflect that. A two-hour half-marathon is the race I am running into.

THE GRIT DOCTOR SAYS:

You ran it in 2 hours 1 minute Ruth. Bad luck. You lost.

RUNNING A MARATHON IS NOT REALLY ABOUT RUNNING A MARATHON

When you're out on your fourth run of the week, pounding the streets through the lashing rain and with a new blister ripening on your heel, it helps to remember that there are upsides to training for a marathon. Massive upsides ...

So what is it all about, then?

You may have entered your first marathon – as I did – for no reason other than being up for a challenge. If, like me, you were not a runner when you signed up, you may also be slightly mad and certainly not expecting to hear what I am about to say: by the time you actually run your marathon you will be running it in celebration of the person that you have become through the process of training for it, *because running a marathon is not really about running a marathon.* It is about all the shitty runs you have nailed, all the sacrifices you have made, and all that your body and mind has endured over many months to get you to that starting line, primed and ready to win. Running regularly has already impacted the rest of your life; helped organise your eating, weight, time-keeping and moods! No doubt you've noticed all sorts of other unexpected benefits too. Well, the marathon will catapult you into a new sphere of being because it is the very pinnacle, the apex and the epicentre of all you have learnt and experienced.

The marathon transforms your body and soul into that of a champion, of someone who has proven to themselves that they can overcome all the odds, of someone who can laugh in the face of defeat and push past it, of someone who embraces all their pain – mental and physical – and who faces their biggest fears and powers through them all regardless. In taking this on, you will become the very best version of yourself and the knock-on effect is unreal. And it doesn't just come from crossing the finishing line, it comes gradually through the discipline you acquire over the gruelling training schedule that you will somehow manage to fit into this crazily busy life of yours. It will remodel your body and make you supremely efficient; your body learning to enjoy being worked in a way it has never experienced, and your mind, as if by magic and in profound gratitude, also operating in an inspired running-induced utopia.

Time travel

People are so often put off entering a marathon because they believe that the time commitments will have a negative impact on the rest of their lives. But here's a secret no one tells you: when you are training for a marathon, an extraordinary thing will happen to your experience of time. You actually *win time* through training. Unbelievable though that must sound, your training plan will force you to become superhuman, capable of multi-tasking at a level you have only ever dreamed of. The time you invest in your training is not eating into your 24-hour daily quota – if the miles you run were being put into a time bank, you would get a greater return the more miles you invested. This is the best thing about doing a marathon – what it brings to the rest of your life. This is why people – ordinary people – keep coming back to do another one. In challenging yourself to something so extreme, in putting yourself out there on the line and committing to something so hard and so visceral, you become a player: powerful and in charge, energetic, efficient and passionate. Running the marathon is one of the ways to become the very best version of yourself – both physically and mentally.

THE GRIT DOCTOR SAYS:
Training wins you time. FACT.

AND NOW FOR SOME MORE GOOD NEWS

Through the process of training for your marathon you will experience some if not all of the following:

- Increased productivity – which means getting more shit done in less time.

- Overall increase in well-being and a more positive outlook on life.

- A better physique – toned and lean.

- A much healthier heart.

- Better sleep and less stress.

- An incredible sense of accomplishment which spills into a new CAN DO attitude to apply to other pursuits.

There are many more benefits that *you* will experience on your own personal marathon journey. And they come not from running the marathon itself but are acquired steadily over the many runs that lead up to it. So treat every training run with respect. Each one is important – the shitty ones, the rainy ones, the easy ones – each one is different but each one is ultimately the same. Every single run brings with it something from the above list and many other benefits too. Every time you are thinking of not going running, of giving up, that it is the worst run ever and that you are hating it more than life itself, remember that it is not just a run, it does not exist in isolation. It is another critical step towards bringing you home, to the finishing line, and to winning.

CHARIDEE AND FUNDRAISING

Most race-runners, from 5kers to marathoners, are sponsored to raise money for charity – it is an incredibly useful motivational tool and only enhances the smug glow of post-race achievement. With marathons it's even more important, both as a tool to keep your training on track and, often, as the only way you can secure a place in the more popular races. In committing to raise money for a charity, you are making a very public statement about your intentions: both to actually run in the race *no matter what* and to raise the

money you have pledged. This can be hugely useful motivating fuel when the sofa is beckoning – bringing to mind
what you have promised and realising with a start how many
people you would be letting down in failing to deliver. This
thought alone ought to have you into your trainers and
punching out a fast six-miler instantly.

THE GRIT DOCTOR SAYS:
It works if you make it work for you.

Turn to the Applying for a Marathon chapter to see how the
London Marathon allocates charity places.

Now, in The Grit Doctor's eyes, all charities were created
equal where the marathon is concerned. This may be a
slightly controversial position (but when has The Grit Doctor
ever shied away from a bit of controversy?) but I have yet to
come across any charity that isn't a worthy enough cause to
run for. One of the fatal traps of first-time marathon running
is biting off more than you can chew charity-wise and thus
getting your knickers in a twist for all the wrong reasons.

So if you want to guarantee your place in the marathon by
running it for a charity and pledging to raise money, which
The Grit Doctor recommends to avoid ballot disappointment, my advice is to find the charity – a small charity –
which requires that you raise the least amount of money.

Why aim so low? Well, contentious though this may seem at first blush, it is far better to have a realistic fund-raising goal that isn't going to stress you out completely and eat into valuable training time. Plus, the smaller charities need your support more. And, you may actually end up raising much more than you set out to anyway. So, it's a win win WIN. You win your place in the marathon, you are supporting and raising awareness for a less well-known and under-funded charity but, most importantly, you are not setting yourself up for a nervous breakdown when you realise a few weeks before race day that you have failed to raise the first £1000 of the £5000 target you committed to.

This is my general advice to first-time marathoners who are on no particular quest, save for taking on the massive personal challenge of running 26.2 miles. Of course there will be those among you whose participation in the marathon is directly linked to a very specific cause, charity or illness, and raising awareness for that cause is not only the driving force behind what you are doing, it is the sole reason for having entered the marathon in the first place. I get it. I applaud and salute you. You may be doing it in fancy dress, you may be spending much more time fund-raising than running and that is absolutely fine by me. Your 'win' may be raising a huge amount of money. (Be sure to declare this as your goal so you are clear what a win is for you.) Whatever your win is, remain focused on it using the motivational sections of this book to help you stay on track.

Begging for money

This is what it always feels like when you do the whip-round via email and social media, especially during the current appalling economic climate when everyone feels more strapped for cash than ever before. Well, almost everyone. Probably everyone we are friends with. There is, however, a group of people who have money that they literally *have* to give away to charity or it goes to the tax man. This money is there for the taking, as it were, and there is plenty of it knocking about in the City and big businesses. So, when begging for money, AIM HIGH. Don't ask your penniless best mate or work colleague, go straight to the MD, the chairman, the CEO, the boss you've never met but whose name is the very company you slave under. They have the money. Perhaps you could ask your company to match any money you raise?

This strategy also means you avoid the dreadful social awkwardness that can come with asking your contemporaries to cough up. Obviously, this doesn't extend to your immediate family, who should always pay on demand and be there on race day to cheer you on.

THE GRIT DOCTOR SAYS:
ASK THE BIG GUNS.

Ruth

A hopeless fundraiser, it has to be said. But when I did the Three Peaks Challenge back in 2004 (walking, not running) I was involved with this incredible group of women – sisters, in fact – who were phenomenally good at fundraising and were incredibly committed to the cause – The Charlie Waller Memorial Trust, which raises awareness of depression, having lost their mother to the illness that Christmas. One of the things they did was organise a party at which we all offered something for auction. Everyone loves a party, and even more so, a party with a purpose. The auction was the purpose in this case, but it could be fancy dress or any theme that provides a focal point. And don't forget, everyone is happier to part with cash after a few drinks. It is all about giving as well as receiving, which is a far more attractive option than the usual dry begging letter/email/tweet and frankly, makes asking for cash infinitely less embarrassing. If you don't have the time or the balls to organise a fundraiser yourself, piggyback onto someone else's (as I did) or think of something you can offer off your own bat. I heard about a fundraiser who is offering baked homemade treats for every fiver donated. Immediate appeal. Genius. I'm in.

There are plenty of ways to sex up your fundraising efforts. www.guess2give.com is a new and frankly ingenious way of raising money in which the giver can also become a prize-winner: The Grit Doctor's clear favourite. For more vanilla fundraising, make the most of sites such as www.justgiving.com and www.virginmoney-giving.com to organise your efforts – so much simpler than the sponsorship forms of yore. At the very least, you can fling the link up on Facebook, sit back and watch your total stack up.

I CAN'T DO IT

There will almost certainly come a time during your marathon training when you'll have to fight an overwhelming urge to quit. It may happen to you more than once. It may happen every week just before you do your long run. The training programme is long and arduous – there's just no way around that – and sustaining your running mojo is going to be tough. So what do you do when the little voice in your head starts whispering that you'll never be able to do it? *You're too weak, too fat, too lazy, too scared, too much of a FAT BITCH.*

This is when your only option is to call upon the techniques you learnt earlier in the book. You may have a devil on your shoulder, but you also have a feisty Inner Bitch who is more than capable of shouting down your tormentor. She was the one who got you up off the sofa in the first place and the one who made you laugh all the way home when you first nailed your circuit. Listen to her again now. Tune into her voice, let her get right up in your face. When you feel like giving up, she will make you soldier on. Go back and read Chapter 2 if you're struggling to locate her. Every single time 'I can't do it' raises its ugly head, her response is an Obama-esque **YES. YOU. CAN.**

THE GRIT DOCTOR SAYS:

Enough fromage. Let the grit begin.

17

EVERY TIME YOU RUN YOU WIN

The key to kicking the marathon's arse is to keep running regularly: *at least* four times a week with a long run every weekend that gets longer and longer until you can run 20 miles. Once you can run 20 miles – and I recommend you only do it once, ideally peaking about three weeks before race day – you've made it. Never underestimate the power of race-day adrenalin and the rush you'll get from the crowd cheering you on through those final untested 6.2 miles. (That 0.2 may well feel like a marathon within the marathon if you have been sabotaged by The Wall.)

The physical and mental strength required to complete those 26.2 miles is enormous and mind over matter can only help you if you have done the necessary training. Without the necessary training, even the grittiest character, with the greatest will in the world, won't have a prayer of completing a marathon running and 'winning' on race day. Your body and mind will simply collapse under the strain.

I've designed a training programme that will get you – with a good dose of grit – race ready. But remember that The Grit Doctor expects you to take responsibility for your own progress and to adapt the plan to suit your own fitness level and lifestyle. If you fancy squeezing an extra weekly run in to your plan, that's great, and will make the job on race day that bit easier. You'll all be coming at this from different levels of fitness, with varying reserves of motivation and with different 'wins' fixed in your mind. Use the tools here to help you figure out how to make the plan work for you.

THE GRIT DOCTOR SAYS:

If you are a marathon aficionado, congrats. I am very flattered that you are reading this. But as you will know, if you want to run a two-and-a-half-hour marathon, you are going to have to run five or six times a week and increase your speed, sprints, hills and midweek mileage too. The plans herein are for first-timers.

Ok, bitches, let's get marathoning.

THE GRIT DOCTOR CALCULATOR

The Grit Doctor Calculator is Step 1, the first thing to do once you've signed up for the race. It will help you work out how to organise your training plan.

THE GRIT DOCTOR SAYS:

The calculator assumes you are running *at least* three times a week for 45 minutes, comfortably.

First, write down the distance you are currently running on your regular, three-times-a-week run. If it's six miles, subtract six from twenty miles – which is the furthest you will run during training – and then add on three-weeks' tapering off time and you will be left with the ideal number of weeks you need to be marathon-ready. (For the half-marathon, subtract your 'comfortable run' distance in miles from twelve miles – the furthest you will run till race day: 12 – 6 + 3.)★

Taking the six-mile example above:

20 – 6 + 3 = 17

+ 6 weeks (contingency)

★Ideally you should give yourself another six weeks (three for the half-marathon) slippage time to allow for any injuries and unforeseen circumstances that may interrupt your training. Both plans expect you to increase your mileage by one mile per week, and give you a huge amount of breathing space for injury time-outs and tapering. Don't let that make you complacent.

So it's 17 weeks of solid training, never missing the long weekend run when you will be adding on the extra mile. If you have to miss a session occasionally, it is not a train-smash provided it is any session other than your long weekend run. Not negotiable.

THE GRIT DOCTOR SAYS:

Your marathon needs to be run within twelve months of your decision to enter it. It would be impossible to sustain your motivation, as well as damaging for you physically, to begin marathon training now for a marathon three years later.

That said, if the calculator tells you that you have a surfeit of time, for the love of God don't curl up on the sofa and practise carb-loading. Start training NOW. Use the extra time to push yourself further and adjust your 'win' accordingly. You will be very glad for that extra time because as race day approaches, you will *always* wish that you had more time and that you had trained harder. This is a good thing by the way, wishing you had done more. It means that you give a shit, that you want to win.

THE GRIT DOCTOR SAYS:

You are never going to wake up on race day and think, I wish I'd had less time to train for this.

What if there's not enough time to train for the marathon I signed up for?

Be sensible. If you are a few weeks or a month short, and feel up to it, you can always add on an extra half-mile or mile to your weekend run and speed up your programme that way. You may of course get lucky and not need to utilise all of your slippage time. Just be realistic and prudent. If you have never run before, and entered a marathon that is just two months away, you may have to completely re-evaluate your expectations and work out what a 'win' will realistically be for you *for this race*. It may be just getting round the course in one piece – walking if necessary. You can still participate in the marathon but there is no way around the lack of training. The marathon is rigorous, demanding and there are absolutely no short cuts to getting your body in a position where it is capable of running the full distance. Don't think, like I did, that because you are young and have previously been really sporty you don't need to do all the training. Everybody does. No exceptions. Walk it this time (or jog/walk) and commit to signing up for the same race next year. AND NAILING IT.

Ruth

I recently ran a 10k in Wexford and decided during the race that I'd like to run a half-marathon. I planned a couple of short easy runs the week I got back to London and my first longish run the following weekend. It was not to be. I was thwarted by an enormous blood-blister which formed under the big toenail on my right foot during the race – there was no chance I was going to be able to run that week. I required minor surgery to remove the gammy nail, which the blister had split, and my doc said no running for three weeks. This is the longest break I've had from running since I started up again about a year ago and, guess what? I've caught a cough, cold and conjunctivitis to boot. I am like a walking Frankenstein with a seeping gammy toe at one end and a seeping gammy eye at the other. Thank God I don't have to see anyone.

LESSONS LEARNED

Factor in unexpected injuries and unforeseen life events that may interrupt training in a big way. Not only did I lose three weeks of training when I lost my toenail, it took another six or seven runs, after starting up again, until I felt back to my old self. Remember that the main thing with the marathon is to keep running regularly – four times a week minimum including a long run every weekend. The long run at the weekend is the key to your marathon success, but **adaptability is also vital. If you have to miss a long weekend run, then swap one of your other sessions during the week for it.** Religiously sticking to a precise schedule can be limiting – you need to remember that provided you are putting in the miles and going on a long run every week, you are on track. Adjust your programme to suit your lifestyle (and to accommodate blips that injury/illness create) because we are all subject to random quirks that can affect our running mojo. There may be days when, thanks to injury or illness, you can't run. There will be other days when, because of rain, periods, families, whatever, running feels like the last thing you want to do. Those are the days when you have to summon your Inner Bitch and run through it. But there will also be days when you'll get sudden bursts of enthusiasm and energy that can spur you on to go further and faster than ever. One day, for no apparent reason, you may wake up full of beans and feel like you could squeeze in an extra-long run or simply must conquer that hill. If this happens to you, for goodness sake, DO IT, irrespective of what your 'programme' is telling you to do that day.

TRAINING HOME TRUTHS

- Accept that a punishing training regime is a MUST. Start to see 'punishing' as compulsory medicine necessary for success on race day.

- Take on the fact that the training will be HARD. At times it will be CONFRONTING. It will also be CHALLENGING, not just physically but mentally too.

- There will be many a training run that your brain and body refuse to comply with. YOU RUN IT ANYWAY. Every run, especially a bad one, is another run out of the way, another run done, another step closer to the finishing line. Much like contractions in childbirth, each one is bringing you closer to home ... so my Irish grandmother used to say, and she had 10 children!

- Many of your runs will be unbelievably BORING.

- And accept that embracing all of the above is about PLUCK.

THE GRIT DOCTOR SAYS:
Pluck it up.

TIME-MANAGEMENT TIPS

- **Fit training runs around your existing schedule** – so to or from work (that rucksack will have proven to be a valuable grit add-on come race day) or very early mornings and early evenings for mums currently at home with children.

- If, like me, you are at home working or with babies or small children all week (and aren't too vain), **get dressed in your running kit** when you wake up in the morning. That way you are always run-ready whenever the chance might present itself during the day – and you have an excuse for wearing jogging bottoms every day.

- **Get your run done** and out of the way at the first available opportunity. That way, you won't waste any time worrying about not yet having done it, but more importantly, you will reap the benefits for a greater part of the day, putting those post-run endorphins to work for you in the rest of your day's activities, whether you're at work or at home.

- **Be organised with meals**. If you are using an evening slot to run, after you're home from work/the babies are down, plan and prepare your evening meal before you go so it is ready, or almost ready, when you get back. I make large quantities of chilli con carne, for example, which I freeze in portions and defrost that morning. I stick a couple of potatoes in the oven just before I go off running and by the time I'm home, dinner's ready. Getting really anal with your meal planning will pay dividends in terms of time management.

- **Do your long run at the weekend.** *There is always time.* Those of you with babies/toddlers, use their lunchtime nap for runs or early evenings when they have gone to bed. Begging your other half to look after them while you go off running may become a bit punchy as your runs take you past the two-hour mark, especially if you have twin toddlers. Don't punish your other half for your training schedule. Go about your training with such uncompromising fairness and commitment that it adds to and doesn't detract from your relationship.

THE GRIT DOCTOR SAYS:

Get your run done *at the very first* opportunity each training day.

INTERVALS

Ruth

I've realised that one of the major things holding me back as a runner is my uncanny ability to always dodge a fartlek (the fancy – Swedish – name for interval training) session. It was only when I was comprehensively thrashed by my younger sister when we ran together recently and she told me about the interval training she does every Tuesday (location: Primrose Hill; drill: sprint up hill to first lamppost against someone a little bit fitter and faster than her; jog down, sprint up to second lamppost and then jog all the way back down; sprint up to third lamppost and jog all the way down, and repeat until you reach the top ... half dead) that I experienced first-hand the impact of committed interval/hill training. Note how her fartlek training session is done on a very steep hill so she is combining the two best things to improve stamina (hills and sprints!) with endurance and speed in the one session. Talk about time-savvy. Doing this every week, it is hardly surprising that she can nail a 10k race in 44 minutes and is forever saying to me towards the end of a run together, when I am on my knees, 'Let's give it a nudge', before she flies off leaving a trail of dust in her wake.

You can get away without any interval training at 5k and 10k, possibly even the half-marathon (although your performances would undoubtedly be vastly improved, especially in the latter two categories, if you did), but you cannot avoid it if your marathon goal is to finish in a competitive time.

Ruth

It's 31 May and I've just got back from a run. Not as hot and sweaty as the previous three this week – it felt easy. For the first time and as a way of a gentle re-introduction to fartlek, I simply told myself towards the end of the run to sprint for 50 seconds (counting to 50 in my head – no faffing about with fancy watches required), then I jogged very slowly to recover for 50 seconds. Then I sprinted again for 60 seconds and recovered for 50 seconds. Then 70 seconds sprint/50 seconds recovery. Next time I am going to start at sprinting for 70/50 then build up to 80, then 90. I almost enjoyed it – there was something incredibly exhilarating and a little bit frightening about truly sprinting again, letting my legs stretch out fully. It was a celebration of the strength in my legs and the distinct lack of pain in my knees or anywhere else for that matter.

NEXT UP: CORE STRENGTH

Running has become so much more difficult for me since I had the twins, and I think one of the reasons – aside from general fatigue – is that my middle, my core, has lost a lot of tone since having a C-section. It is patently clear that improving our core strength will most certainly improve our running performance *and* help guard against injury. Sounds like a pretty crucial component of marathon training to me.

The Grit Doctor is a lifelong fan of the simple sit-up and I began doing them again recently: 3 sets of 20 reps with 30 seconds rest between reps. I am in AGONY the next day, but a good sort of agony – I know I used those muscles good and proper. And running seems to loosen them up again nicely.

How to sit-up

To do a basic sit-up properly, lie down with your legs spread to about shoulder-width apart, knees bent and feet on the floor. Put your hands by your ears and elbows out to the sides – your hands are not supposed to pull you up at all, your core is. Look straight ahead, chin off your chest to keep your neck relaxed (you don't want to be developing neck muscles – it's not a good look). Place the small of your back into the floor and using your core, breathe in and lift your shoulders neck and head off the ground to about 30 degrees, hold for a second or two and then breathe out and return to the starting position. Easy. Repeat up to 20 times *if you are able*. But be realistic. If you have never done a sit-up before this may be difficult, so don't try and run before you can walk. The key to this exercise is smooth, slow movements where all the effort is felt in your abdomen. Don't be put off if your stomach seems to swell up initially (mine looks enormous today). It is just readjusting itself to being used again having been in a coma for years. The last time I had to adopt a similar position and felt my abdomen contract was during labour, and so with each sit-up I thank God I'm not having a contraction. It makes the 20 reps feel like a walk in the park ...

THE MARATHON BORE

You know who you are. You have begun to talk *at* people, to talk about the carbohydrate content of what you are eating as if it is quite normal chat. Obsessively thinking in miles and kilometres and again, carbs, AND TALKING ABOUT IT INCESSANTLY. There is much about marathon training that will change you and it is all good. BUT IT IS NOT GOOD TO TALK ABOUT IT ALL THE TIME. Just because you are running a marathon does not make you in any way more interesting than the next person. You have learnt incredible physical discipline through your gruelling training runs, now use it to exercise some bloody mental discipline. That means no matter how strong the urge to bang on about your last 15-miler, SHUT THE F★★★ UP instead. You give running marathons a bad name.

It is also worth mentioning that your other half should not be made to suffer unnecessarily on account of your marathon exploits. That means no banging on to them about the above either. Exercise some restraint and be respectful. Simple things like not leaving your stinking running clothes and trainers lying around the house pay dividends. If you continue to insist on doing your long run during bath time on a Sunday evening, while your other half deals with your brood of toddlers, don't be surprised if instead of turning up on race day to cheer you on, they use the time to pack up and move out.

HALF-MARATHON TRAINING PLAN

This plan takes up where the 10k training programme left off. It assumes you have completed a 10k race (6.2 miles) recently and relatively comfortably. If you have not you will obviously need longer to prepare for the half-marathon: just use The Grit Doctor Calculator to work out how long you will need and rearrange your training plan accordingly.

THE GRIT DOCTOR SAYS:

Stop asking for a prescription for everything. Start *owning* your training plan, and create it for yourself. The keys to success are: mixing up your pace, taking on the odd hill and never EVER skiving on your long weekend run.

WEEK 1

Monday

Gentle exercise other than running: cross-training, swim, cycle, walk and tuck into some core-strengthening exercises.

Tuesday

Interval training. Incorporate bursts of sprinting into your 40–45-minute run (roughly 3 miles).

Wednesday

40–45 minutes easy running (roughly 3 miles).

Thursday

Rest day.

Friday

Interval training/hill running for 40–45 minutes. Some sprints and some hill action please – fantastically good for improving stamina and endurance.

Saturday

Rest day.

Sunday

Long run – 7 miles.

THE GRIT DOCTOR SAYS:

Don't EVER expect to think 'Whoopy-do, it's interval training day!' Just grit them out and focus on how much easier they're making your long weekend runs.

WEEK 2

Monday As per Week 1.

Tuesday As per Week 1 but try to lengthen the sprints.

Wednesday As per Week 1 but increase the distance by about half a mile.

Thursday As per Week 1.

Friday As per Week 1 but try to lengthen the sprints/the hill or the speed at which you take them on – or both if you are in a grit-tastic kind of mood.

Saturday REST.

Sunday Long run – 8 miles.

THE GRIT DOCTOR SAYS:

You can swap sessions at will, but try not to run on three consecutive days and do not take two consecutive rest days.

WEEK 3

Monday As per Week 1.

Tuesday As per Week 1 but try to reduce recovery times and increase sprinting times. Increase overall distance by about half a mile.

Wednesday As per Week 2.

Thursday REST.

Friday As per Week 1 but trying to reduce recovery times and increasing the number of sprints. Or nail that hill.

Saturday REST.

Sunday Long run – 9 miles.

WEEK 4

Monday As per Week 1.

Tuesday As per Week 1 but more long sprints, shorter recovery jogs when possible. Increase overall distance by roughly half a mile.

Wednesday As per Week 3 but increase overall distance by about half a mile.

Thursday REST.

Friday As per Week 1 but more long sprints, shorter recovery jogs and/or hill training. Push yourself on the sprints.

Saturday REST.

Sunday Long run – 10 miles – with the second half at your half-marathon pace.

THE GRIT DOCTOR SAYS:

If you are running into a timed win, you need to practise running into that time on your long weekend run.

WEEK 5

Monday As per Week 1.

Tuesday As per Week 1 but really extending yourself on the sprints, and sustaining them for longer. Half a mile up on the previous week.

Wednesday As per Week 1.

Thursday REST.

Friday As per Week 1 but really extending yourself on the sprints and/or hill/s!

Saturday REST.

Sunday Long run – 11 miles. Try to run this at your race pace.

THE GRIT DOCTOR SAYS:

Expect to have some shockingly bad weeks during training, and suck them up.

WEEK 6

Monday As per Week 1.

Tuesday As per Week 1. Push yourself on the sprints – you should be really feeling your progress now – and up the distance another half-mile from the previous week (now roughly 5 miles).

Wednesday As per previous week but increase the distance by about half a mile.

Thursday REST.

Friday As per Week 1 and really go for it on the sprints.

Saturday REST.

Sunday Long run – 12 miles. Try to run this at your race pace.

WEEK 7 – tapering

Monday As per Week 1.

Tuesday As per Week 1. Sprints should be second nature by now – a pleasurable twice-weekly grit add-on.

Wednesday As per Week 1 – 45 minutes easy running.

Thursday REST.

Friday 45 minutes easy running, taking on a hill – sorry, what hill?

Saturday REST.

Sunday Long run – 9 miles.

WEEK 8

Monday As per Week 1.

Tuesday As per Week 1 but shorten the number of sprints both in length and number. 45 minutes (roughly 3 miles).

Wednesday As per Week 1 – 45 minutes easy running.

Thursday REST.

Friday As per Week 1 but shorten the number of sprints and really GO FOR IT/take on one small hill AS FAST AS YOU CAN. 45 minutes running in total.

Saturday REST.

Sunday Long run – 8 miles at half-marathon pace.

WEEK 9

Do a couple of short easy runs at half-marathon pace, rest well, and eat plenty of carbs (70% of your plate). Get pumped about race day. Try not to run for the few days before your half-marathon.

MARATHON TRAINING PLAN

Use the half-marathon training plan if you have entered a marathon having recently completed a 10k race and/or are running comfortably at least three times a week for 45 minutes. When you get to the end of Week 6 and have run 12 miles, for Week 7 use the same half-marathon plan during the week but add on an extra mile to your weekend run, taking you to 13 miles. Then instead of going to Week 8, skip to Week 1 of the Marathon Plan.

If you are entering a marathon having just completed a half-marathon, you should be ready, according to The Grit Doctor Calculator, in another 10 weeks: $20 - 13 + 3$ (tapering) $= 10$ (plus slippage time). The Grit Doctor Calculator is a most generous and forgiving machine, because there is nothing more stressful than not having enough time to do yourself justice. Use The Grit Doctor Calculator and plans as your skeleton programme from which to create a training programme to suit yourself.

WEEK 1

Monday
Cross-training: cycle, swim, walk, ride and do some core-strengthening exercises. Grit out some sit-ups. Remember The Grit Doctor's position on Mondays. Do not bring on a Mondageddon. If you did do your long run on the Sunday

this *must* be taken as a rest day. Your long runs are now of such a length that you need to rest your muscles the following day or risk compromising your training and increasing the likelihood of injury. And you will reap the psychological rewards from Sunday's long run all day at work while your legs are enjoying a well-deserved rest under the desk.

Tuesday
Fartlek/interval training. Incorporate bursts of sprinting into your roughly 5.5-mile run.

Wednesday
40–45 minutes easy running.

Thursday
REST.

Ruth

I am using the same circuit for all my runs other than my longer weekend run and even then I am incorporating my usual run at the beginning. Is this unbelievably boring? Yep, and boring is just how I like it. Boring frees me up to think about other stuff. Plus, it reduces the amount of time I think about where I might run to, which reduces the risk I might change my mind while planning and procrastinating over where to go, and I am convinced it minimises injury from falling as I know the course so well:

I could run it blindfolded. None of it is on concrete which is a huge plus, the canopy provided by the trees shields me from the sun's rays and the rain, it is pretty enough to keep me interested but familiar enough to allow my thoughts to wander, and there is the odd hill and gentle incline which, on fartlek days, I am sprinting through.

Friday

Interval/hill running for 40–45 minutes. Some sprints and some uphill.

Saturday

REST.

If your win is a timed win – i.e. you plan to complete the race under a certain time – you need to run some of your long runs at goal pace. This means working out what your time per mile needs to be in order that you complete the marathon within the time you have set yourself. I.e. if you want to run a four-hour marathon that translates to nine-minute miles. This will get you used to that pace so it becomes second nature and once the runs get very long, you can run the first half slower and then the second part at marathon pace, which gets your body used to upping the pace when it really doesn't want to. Your weekday runs are about improving your speed and endurance and stamina to tackle the longer weekend run which is, mile by mile, preparing you and moulding you for race day.

Sunday

Long run – 14 miles.

THE GRIT DOCTOR SAYS:

The key to marathon success is running your race at a consistent pace.

WEEK 2

As per Week 1 but increase the length of your Tuesday interval run by roughly half a mile and push yourself speed-wise on your Friday 45-minute interval/hill run. Extend your long run at the weekend by one mile to 15 miles (run at least the second half at marathon pace if you have a goal time in mind).

WEEK 3

As per Week 1 but increase the length of your Tuesday interval run by roughly half a mile (up from the previous week to 6.5 miles) and your long run at the weekend by a mile to 16 miles (run at least the second half at marathon pace).

THE GRIT DOCTOR SAYS:

I hate recommending buying 'kit'. If you have a watch, use it to keep you running at a

consistent race pace. If you don't, buy one if
you feel the need.*

WEEK 4

As per previous week but increase the length of your long
run at the weekend by a mile to 17 miles (run at least the
second half at marathon pace).

THE GRIT DOCTOR SAYS:

During your long runs, pay close attention to
what your body is saying. Notice when your
muscles start to feel *really* tired – breaking-
point tired – and if and when your brain goes
foggy. These are warning signs that The Wall is
imminent. The more you are in tune with the
signs of chronic fatigue during those long
practice runs, the better equipped you will be
on race day to deal with them. Practise
speeding up when you are truly knackered;
practise with gels, energy drinks, chocolate and

---

* I am not buying a special running watch for my half-marathon training, I
am just using my common sense and a clock I pass on my run. Thankfully,
some races have pacemakers carrying balloons/signs for runners to check
what finishing time they are running into. That's sufficient for me. Or ask a
fellow runner with all the gadgets as you overtake him.

sweets to see what works to give you an energy boost when you need it most.

WEEK 5

As per previous week but increase the length of your Tuesday interval run by roughly half a mile to 7 miles and your long run at the weekend by a mile to 18 miles (run at least the second half at marathon pace).

THE GRIT DOCTOR SAYS:

Get out of the habit of 'treating' yourself and get into the habit of considering it to be a treat that you are able to train for and participate in a marathon. IT IS THE TREAT.

WEEK 6

As per previous week but increase your pace on the sprints and hill/s on Tuesday's and Thursday's interval sessions and your long run at the weekend by a mile to 19 miles (run at least the second half at marathon pace).

THE GRIT DOCTOR SAYS:

Your long runs are all dress rehearsals for the big day.

WEEK 7

As per Week 1 (go easy during the week to prepare for the biggie at the weekend) but increase your long run at the weekend by a mile to 20 miles (run at least the second half at marathon pace). **This is it – you will not run further than this until race day. Congratulations on nailing the longest run of your life.**

WALL IT

THE GRIT DOCTOR SAYS:

Embrace The Wall. If you don't get even a whiff of her during your marathon you have not been running hard enough.

You are going to hear about 'The Wall' a lot during your training. You may meet her during your marathon some-where after the 20-mile mark. And she is not going to be your new best friend. The key to your success on race day is man-aging WHEN you meet The Wall, not IF you meet her. Fearing The Wall too much may cause you not to push your-self hard enough, but not treating her with something approaching reverential respect may mean she destroys all your chances of winning. The Wall is a place where your body meets its breaking point, where there is nothing left in the tank, the glycogen reserves stored up in your muscles have been spent in getting you this far and your central nervous system is going into meltdown. It is a place of total mental and physical exhaustion where every fibre of your being is telling you to give up. That you can't do it. BUT. YOU. CAN.

A GRIT DOCTOR ANALOGY:

Think of your marathon race as a game between you and The Wall. You will win the race if you outsmart your opponent.

But how?

1. Make sure you don't see her before the 20-mile mark. The best safeguard against this happening is having trained properly (especially on those long weekend runs which are essential for Wall-management) and having eaten and rested well the week before. If you meet her too early on, she **will** break you.

2. **Know your enemy**. Start to recognise the signs of intense fatigue on your long training runs and practise outsmarting them. **Work out what works** – try a glucose drink or gel on a long run and see if that helps.

3. Just when you sense she is coming (and assume from mile 20 onwards that she is there, just a few hundred yards ahead in the distance), go into **RUN FAT**

BITCH RUN mode: in other words, **speed up** – those fast-twitch muscle fibres may still have some glycogen remaining in them, having not been used thus far at your slower marathon-running pace. Use them now, they may see you through a mile or so.

4. Create a faux emergency situation in your brain – **GRIT-MANIA:** tell yourself **I WILL** pass that man in front of me in the banana suit **at any cost**. Get angry, get aggressive (inside that is, don't go lashing out at him and end up getting yourself arrested during the closing stages of the race). What I mean is, channel it: ALL your rage, ALL your hunger, ALL your passion, ALL your pain, ALL your hatred. If you have been practising getting gritty with yourself during your long training runs, this should prove to be no problem at all. It may just enable you to override your central nervous system and power through for another mile or so.

THE GRIT DOCTOR SAYS:

None of this will work if you have gone careering headlong into The Wall completely unawares. As soon as you pass the 20-mile mark and feel an *overwhelming* urge to stop in a way you haven't experienced thus far, assume it to be The Wall, *and then, just before you meet her, NAIL her.*

WEEK 8

As per Week 1 but keep the length of your interval/hill runs the same and decrease the length of your long run at the weekend by 3 miles to 17 miles.

WEEK 9

One short interval/hill run (45 minutes) early in the week and two short easy runs on other days of your choosing. Decrease the length of your long run by 4 miles to 13 miles but run it all at your marathon pace.

WEEK 10

As per Week 1 but only one interval/hill run towards the beginning of the week and two short easy runs with two days off before marathon day. Use these days for some core-strength training and much pasta and pie eating (throughout the day, not face-stuffing just before bed-time).

THE GRIT DOCTOR SAYS:
This week is for filling your motivation tank alongside your carb tank.

While devouring pies as though your life depends on it, fill your brain with lots of motivation stuff, re-read anything in this book that has inspired you, listen to motivating music, memorise motivating mantras and themes that really work for you. How do you know if it works? If it gives you shivers down your spine when you bring it to mind, it is definitely one for the memory bank. Check out stuff on YouTube, have a good laugh too and get yourself in the mood for winning. Read, relax, focus and get excited about race day. May the Grit be with us . . .

For more tips on race-day strategies and advice on how to prepare for the big day, turn to Chapter 19.

THE GRIT DOCTOR SAYS:

Now that you are here – race day – it is not the taking part that counts. From here on in, it's all about winning.

18

NUTRITION – CARB-ORAMA

THE GRIT DOCTOR SAYS:

Training for and running a marathon puts enormous strain on your body. Its demands can only be met through *nourishment not punishment.*

The Grit Doctor does not want you to spend too much time fussing over food. A lot of valuable training time can be wasted by analysing your diet and planning overly complicated carb-ratio-precise meals. You are already eating *relatively* well, having devoured the rest of the book and hopefully abiding by its simple rules *most of the time.* Of course it is important to be mindful of what you're putting into your body, but provided you aim to eat a diet made up of at least 55% carbohydrate, you won't go far wrong.

THE GRIT DOCTOR SAYS:

You really don't have to watch what you eat *in terms of your weight.* But you do need to watch what you eat in terms of your running performance.

The main thing about marathon running is that you can massively relax the eating guidelines laid down previously. The Golden Rules remain but I have added a third – DRINK. *EVEN. MORE.* WATER. Your water intake must reflect the significant increase in your weekly mileage. You don't have to stick to plain water either. I have been drinking gallons of VERY WEAK lemon barley and loads of Earl Grey tea. Caffeine is a perfectly acceptable stimulant for marathon training and I find an espresso before a run can be just the ticket to get me through those awful first ten minutes. Others swear by isotonic sports drinks and gels. I think they are revolting.

As well as upping your H_2O intake, this section will be a real celebration of the carb – the fuel that will help you get through those gruelling 26.2 miles.

The more miles you run, the more fuel you need in the tank. And the better quality the fuel, the smoother your engine will run. So it's all about making sure the food you are eating is delivering what you need to nourish that hard-working body of yours.

Some **Grit Doctor pointers** to help keep you on track:

1. **Listen** to your body. When we really listen to our bodies we *know* what it is we need. Running makes the voice of your body much easier to hear.

THE GRIT DOCTOR SAYS:
In training for a marathon your body will start to tell you what it wants you to put into it.
Practise obedience.

---

2. The most important aspect to your diet is: **common sense**. 'But, but, but ... don't I need to eat certain types of carbs?' True, to a degree, and I have devised a very simple test to demonstrate just how good your common sense is in this very regard.

3. **Treats** can be had when you fancy them **(WITHIN REASON)**, although don't be gorging on a tub of ice-cream or a roast dinner just before setting out on an interval training session. Be sensible, and eat loads of good carbs *at the right times*. You will get to learn what your body runs best on during the course of your training programme.

4. Eat your main meal *after* your training run (within an

hour or so of completing it). **Do not eat a main meal before a run**, especially a big one. Leave plenty of time (two hours at least) after eating a meal, whether it's breakfast, lunch or dinner, before setting out on a run.

5. Do eat a **carby snack** half an hour before a run if you fancy one, and whether you fancy one or not, *always* eat something carby before a long run – some whole-meal toast, a bowl of cereal, a banana, that sort of thing.

6. Take a few chunks of **chocolate** or half a Snickers bar on a really long run (over 10 miles) if you think you might need it and the prospect of eating it halfway through really spurs you on.

7. You will need to **take water on long runs**, as well as energy gels/energy sweets/energy bars if that's your thing.

8. **Exercise some self-control**: the leaner you are, the easier the marathon will be to run – lugging around all that excess weight is only going to hold you back because only you can carry it. So, if you've entered a marathon in a moment of madness and are really over-weight, focus on reducing the excess alongside your training plan by EATING. LESS. CRAP.

9. **Don't ignore proteins** in your quest to become a carb queen. Lean meats, fish, eggs and cheese are the obvious sources of good protein and are essential for replenishing

iron stores and building muscle. But it's the carb that must dominate the plate.

THE GRIT DOCTOR SAYS:

Don't panic. It is easy to get into the habit of looking at a plate of food and judging with your eye if it is roughly balanced.

And yes, you are right. Not all carbs were created equal. Good carbs are basically low-GI carbs – the glycemic index classifies how quickly and how much the carbohydrate concerned raises blood sugar levels when compared to pure glucose. (Now now, don't nod off just yet.) Think of low-GI carbs as good carbs because they release their energy slowly. Slow release is the answer to every long-distance runner's needs for the very obvious reason that you require your energy levels to be sustained over a long period of time. GOOD carbs are very easy to spot if you apply your own common sense. I have devised this simple carb-test for you:

Which is the better carb?

- Wholemeal rye toast or white sliced

- Cornflakes or bran flakes

- White rice or brown rice

- Ryvita or chocolate hobnob

- Crisps or jacket potato

- Fresh vegetables or a processed vegetarian ready-meal

If you didn't get all these right within ten seconds flat, you are beyond salvation, I'm afraid. When we think of carby foods: Pasta, Bread, Potatoes, Cereals and Rice all spring to mind (**PBPCR**s – sounds like membership of an incredibly important international organisation. Try to commit this to memory). These – the **PBPCR**s – are all fantastically good carby foodstuffs around which to base your meals, but you should always try to choose the brown version (wholemeal/wholewheat) rather than the processed white variety. (Except when it comes to pasta. Brown pasta has no place on God's earth.) Fruit, vegetables, beans and pulses are also good news, in that they contain good carbohydrate, but in smaller quantities than the **PBPCR**s. In running terms, this means you will get less energy from them to fuel your runs; less bang for your buck. However, what they lack in energy-giving qualities, they make up for in vitamins and fibre and can be eaten by the truckload.

THE GRIT DOCTOR SAYS:

Base your meals around the PBPCRs and you won't go far wrong.

If you must sin, do it after a run and not beforehand. If you fancy a Chinese takeaway or a curry, and let's face it, sometimes only a Domino's pizza will do, the best time to eat it is *after* your long weekend run. In fact, I recommend doing this from time to time, especially if it is just the thing you need to motivate you to get out there on a cold Sunday afternoon and the only thing pushing you up that hill is the thought of an extra slice of Pepperoni Passion . . .

There is **no need** to get bogged down in anything complicated with your eating. Just up your water and 'good carb' intake as you increase your mileage and you'll be fine. You must also incorporate healthy snacks into your diet, especially on training days and most especially on long run training days. Where snacking was not encouraged before, it is quite the opposite with marathon training. Snacking is essential. Snacking is the answer.

A GRIT DOCTOR HEALTH WARNING:

Do not 'DIET' when training for a marathon.

If you are:

An overeater/undertrainer

This is quite common among first-time marathoners and most definitely happened to me. I ate way more than was necessary, fuelled in part by a misguided notion that now I was running four times a week I would waste away unless I trebled my food intake. I completely overdid the eating and as you have already learnt, underdid the training. If you fall into this category – other than the obvious *step up your training* – LISTEN TO YOUR BODY. If it isn't telling you it is hungry, don't eat. Don't pre-empt its signals and stuff your face in a panic because you are going on a six-mile run for the first time. Your body will let you know when it is hungry and when it is full. Learn to trust it.

THE GRIT DOCTOR SAYS:

Trust your body, listen to it carefully and give it what it needs.

An undereater/overtrainer

If you fall into this category, you are going to lose. Anyone who enters the marathon in a misguided and deranged attempt to lose weight and starves themselves while training excessively is doing something incredibly dangerous and potentially life-threatening. You will not be able to cope physically with the demands of training, your heart could fail and your muscles will waste away as they will be eaten to burn as fuel. If you have or may have an eating disorder of any description (other than of the 'I am a fat bitch and eat too much cake' variety), then you must seek medical help for your condition and please do not attempt to train and run a marathon until you are well enough. Indeed, if you have a friend in this position, or notice that someone who was never fat in the first place and in training for a marathon is looking too thin, do try and establish if they have an eating problem and help them to help themselves.

THE GRIT DOCTOR SAYS:
Your body will eat itself. Seek help.

An overeater/overtrainer

You should be fine. Greedy for all things, you are eating as though your life depends on it and training just as hard so oughtn't have any real problems. You are unlikely to change much weight-wise during training (people who eat normally and train properly will invariably lose some weight). The caveat here is that your overeating must be – generally speaking – of good food and not the sinful variety or it may impact negatively on your training and affect your performance on race day.

THE GRIT DOCTOR SAYS:
Work hard. Play hard. Love it.

An undereater/undertrainer

You shouldn't be doing this, and cannot win. The marathon cannot be run on a vicious starvation diet and you are unable to train sufficiently as a result of your daily calorie deficit. There is simply not enough fuel in the tank to run on. You are stuck in a vicious cycle and may well have an eating disorder. Seek medical help and don't attempt to train for and participate in a marathon until you are well enough to cope with the food side of things. Dieting has no part in training and participating in a marathon.

THE GRIT DOCTOR SAYS:
You will lose. Seek professional help.

SAVE THE BEST FOR LAST

The week before the marathon: carb-LOAD. How I love this expression, it's right up there with the word 'pluck' in my book. Loosely translated, it means relax, put your feet up and stuff your face. I recommend alternating pie days with pasta days. You are quite literally loading up with carbs to store up enough glycogen in your muscles, hopefully to keep you going to the finishing line. So it's compulsory binge eating. Sort of. You need to up the carb content of your meals/daily intake to 70–75% which is why it is called *loading*. So, lots of pasta and pie, yes, but at meal times. And for goodness' sake, don't over-indulge to such an extent that you make yourself sick. Death by carb is not the aim of the game.

19

RACE DAY

REDUCING THE WORRY FACTOR

You are in the marathon who you are in life. If you are a born worrier, accept that you will be nervous before the race and take steps to reduce this as much as possible by familiarising yourself with the practical details of the race and planning a timetable for the day (and the days leading up to 'the day') as much as you can. If you're more of a fly-by-the-seat-of-your-pants sort of person, make sure you know where and when the race starts, eat properly and get a good night's sleep. You'll be fine.

- Eat a big pasta dish/nourishing meal/marathon PIE the night before. And if you are the sort of person who worries a lot about this sort of thing, reduce the anxiety by eating a tried-and-tested pre-race meal – i.e. nothing likely to give you an upset stomach. Race day is all about reducing the worry factor. Try it out a few weeks before or as many times as you wish as your evening meal the night before a very long run.

- Finish your breakfast at least three hours before the start of the race.

- Do drink tea, coffee, water or squash up to an hour before the start. I, for one, like a caffeine hit before a race.

- Don't drink your body weight in fluids half an hour before the start, or you'll be wetting yourself when the starting gun fires. If you need a wee mid-race, either do a Paula Radcliffe and just do it, or stop and go. There are Portaloos set up for this during the London Marathon and most well-organised races. It is not a train smash if you have to stop to pee (or even for a number two), as you will be able to start up again and your legs may well thank you for the unexpected short rest.

- If you are aiming to run fast, you should go through a gentle warm-up routine during the 20 minutes leading up to the start – jogging, stretching and striding. You may find you race off quite quickly at the start so your muscles need to be prepared. I am not a big fan of fancy stretches (I don't know how to do them properly)

274

so tend simply to swing my legs up and down while holding onto someone or something and loosen my arm and neck muscles by just shaking myself about a bit. That does it for me.

- Be race-ready. Be sure to have done some race prep in the months leading up to it – 5ks are (I hope?!) a distant memory but the odd 10k and half-marathon race is excellent preparation. You feel differently racing and it gives you a sense of your 'race-day' body and mind. It is similar to an exam in the sense that there is nothing like a set of mocks to get you fired up and to work out what works and what doesn't.

- *You are on your own.* I ran both my marathons with others and found it distracting and the artificial pace-setting unhelpful. I felt as though I was running someone else's marathon on both occasions. This was my choice and I was happy to defer to others because I didn't have the courage to strike out on my own. Next time it will be different.

- Use and abuse other runners/strangers along the way to pace you, to overtake, and to inspire you with tales of courage, but run to your own song from start to finish.

- Do not carry anything during the race, especially not mobile phones, bananas, cameras, etc. If you must carry a drink or snack, find the most lightweight option available that can fit into a zipped pocket and make sure you're used to running with it. There will certainly be drinks stations along the route but I wouldn't bank on getting anything other than good old H_2O. Anything of the energy-giving variety you will need to provide yourself.

- Bring throw-away clothes (or even a bin liner) to keep warm while waiting around and that you can discard at the start or early on in the race. Races usually start early in the morning and there is a considerable amount of waiting around before the race begins. Whatever the forecast, it is likely that you will need some extra layers to begin with. The more disposable these layers are, the better. Again, test this out by participating in races during your training programme so you find out what works best for you, minimising stress levels on race day.

- Lube up. Vaseline your nipples, in between your toes, anywhere that is likely to chafe – believe me, by mile 20 *everything* is starting to chafe. If your thighs meet in the middle (as most normal people's do), lube up there too.

- Do NOT buy and wear new shoes for your race. Do not wear a new outfit either. No amount of Compede or Vaseline will be able to deal with the blisters and burns.

MRS MOTIVATOR

Do have loads of inspiring thoughts, quotes and music – if that's your thing – to keep you motivated and to literally provide shots of adrenalin at the most crucial moments during the race. (I played the *Chariots of Fire* theme tune in my head when I was hitting The Wall and visualised Eric Liddell in the race against Harold Abrahams – when he falls down and you think it's all over, then in brilliant eighties slo-mo, he drags himself up from the floor, rising like a phoenix from the ashes and runs like the wind to the finishing line. It saw me through to the other side.) I have been repeating the line 'Every time you run you win' on training runs, as well as some other mantras – some outlandishly rude and unsuitable for print, others hilarious, others tear-jerkers. Get some of your own and bank them. Something that makes you laugh is also great motivational fuel. Laughing serves several functions: it provides a huge release of pressure, in an instant stops you taking yourself so seriously, and with any luck will give you a much-needed adrenalin shot. There are lots of motivational quotes and videos on my website, www.gritdoctor.com

HOW WILL I FEEL ON RACE DAY?

If you are a control freak and need to know as much as possible about how you will feel and how the day will pan out in meticulous detail, be prepared for a shock. I went through every single emotion that exists on the spectrum of human experience over those 26.2 miles. It was like living an entire lifetime over the course of just one day. In terms of nerves, it was not dissimilar to my wedding day. I was full of nervous anticipation and excitement. The race, much like my wedding, passed by me in a flash and much of the pleasure I derived from it was experienced retrospectively. It is also a bit like childbirth in that no one really talks about the experience of the race itself to the uninitiated because it is almost impossible to explain. It has to be lived through to be understood at all. The truth is that your marathon can only be felt through your own senses, run with your legs and seen through your eyes. Still *have* to know more?

You will have highs, lows, peaks, troughs – as we all do in life. Possibly some agonising pain, hopefully some incomparable joy. Intensely inspiring moments, as well as moments of despair, tears, sweat and possibly blood! Chafing, flatness of emotion, laughter, anger ... the whole frigging lot. And it is EXHAUSTING feeling all this during the space of a few hours, on top of lugging your aching body through 26.2 miles.

The way I dealt with this emotional rollercoaster in

conjunction with the physical exhaustion was to try and focus on the present, on the mile I was running and not to allow myself to think about just how many more miles there were left to run. Taken mile by mile it feels doable, whereas dwelling on the fact you still have 15 miles left can feel a tad overwhelming. I practised a lot of distraction techniques too, looking at the sights, the crowds, listening to other runners' stories en route – anything to stop me focusing on how many more miles I still had to run.

THE GRIT DOCTOR SAYS:
When you have run a really difficult mile, think of it like one of those bad training runs – it is a bad mile out of the way, a bad mile run. Done. Over. A good one is just around the corner waiting to be nailed.

HOW WILL I FEEL AT THE END?

Some people feel completely overwhelmed with emotion as they cross the finishing line and break down in tears. Others, like me, do not. A bit like after a big exam, you may feel incredibly flat in the immediate aftermath. Crossing the finishing line may initially feel like an anti-climax and it is no bad thing to be aware of this and be prepared. But worry not. The real joy, the real glow, the real beauty of the marathon is that you have done it and having done it is going to become a metaphor for you for the rest of your life. A metaphor that says you can achieve anything that you set your mind to provided you put in the effort; a metaphor that speaks for what is possible, for what you are capable of if you just make a commitment to putting one foot in front of the other. And trust me, you will be taking this new-found confidence, this power, into all areas of your life. Where you have felt weak before, you will be stronger; despair, you now know, can be transformed into hope; failure into success. You know that you have to go through all these feelings – good and bad – as part of a necessary process in realising your full potential. You fall down, you pick yourself back up, you are on your knees begging for strength and from nowhere it comes and keeps coming at you in waves. Each and every time you emerge triumphant and stronger than before. You have learnt first-hand that nothing can break the human spirit.

THE GRIT DOCTOR SAYS:

There will be a point during your marathon when you feel as though you are dying. When you will wish you were dead. At some stage following this you will be reborn.

You have done an incredible thing and the magic is just waiting for you in the weeks and months to come. So, in the immediate aftermath, have a nice bath, relax, rehydrate. Don't do what I did and get drunk, nail three Zinger burgers at the counter in KFC and go out dancing till the early hours. (I was young and foolish – and I LOVED it!)

20

RECIPES

I am hugely indebted to my great friends, and fellow runners, Pierce and Marilee Maher of the Potbelly Café in Our Lady's Island, Wexford, and Virginia Marshall of Red Earth Deli in Kingsbridge, Devon, for providing these wonderful recipes.

Pierce's Tagliatelle with Oxtail Ragu

This recipe is *so* simple. Yeah, it takes a few hours to cook but that's what so easy. It can be put in the oven in the morning and by afternoon it's done. Just cook the pasta and that's it.

Ingredients

2 kg oxtail

100 g carrots, finely chopped

100 g celery, finely chopped

100 g onions, finely chopped

4 cloves garlic, finely chopped

4 anchovy fillets

1 tin tomatoes

½ bottle red wine

2 bay leaves

Sprig of rosemary

Sprig of thyme

100 g baby spinach leaves, washed

100 g parmesan

500 ml good beef stock

Salt and black pepper

½ cup flour

Olive oil

1 packet of tagliatelle

A GRIT DOCTOR ASIDE:

Remember Pierce is a top chef and perfectionist: following his recipes to the letter will deliver the ideal pie or pasta dish. But there is no need to panic if, for example, you don't have a sprig of thyme and only a stock cube available. Use your common sense and adapt the recipe where necessary. Obviously, if you don't have the oxtail, you can't make the pasta dish, but not having the rosemary isn't a train-smash for the pie. Common sense please.

Method

Heat olive oil in heavy pot. Coat the oxtail in seasoned flour and fry in olive oil until well browned. Do this in small batches. Remove meat and set aside.

Deglaze the pot with a splash of red wine. Add onions, celery, carrots, anchovy fillets and garlic and fry for five minutes. Add oxtail, tin of tomatoes, beef stock, red wine, bay leaves, rosemary and thyme. Season with salt and pepper and place in pre-heated 140°C oven for 4–5 hours.

Remove from oven; remove bones, herb stalks and bay leaves.

Cook pasta in salted water according to instructions on packet. Drain pasta, leaving some of the cooking water behind. Drizzle with olive oil, add spinach leaves, mix and allow to wilt through pasta.

Spoon pasta into a shallow bowl, spoon oxtail ragu on top. Cover with plenty of grated parmesan.

Try not to eat too quickly and give yourself indigestion. Savour and enjoy!

Pierce's Irish Stew Potbelly Pie

I love Irish stew and I love pies! This recipe combines the two for a wonderful protein- and carb-loaded feast, ideal for people training for a marathon. I've shown how to make hot-water crust pastry, because it's so easy, but if you can't be bothered just use shop-bought pre-rolled pastry – short-crust or puff are both good for this recipe, whichever you prefer.

Ingredients

For the filling:
Vegetable oil
500 g mutton or lamb shoulder cut into 2-inch/
    5 cm chunks
1 kg potatoes, peeled and cut into quarters
115 g onion, roughly chopped
115 g celery, chopped
100 g leeks, cleaned and finely sliced
170 g carrots, roughly chopped
750 ml stock, lamb or chicken
2 bay leaves
Sprig of thyme
Parsley
Salt and pepper
150 g plain flour
For the pastry:

675 g plain flour
255 g salted butter
250 ml whole milk

Method

Heat oil in a heavy frying pan then lightly coat the lamb in seasoned flour and brown off in the pan. Do this in small batches and transfer to a casserole dish.

Fry the onions in the same pan. Before the onions brown, add to casserole dish with meat.

Add the stock, thyme, bay leaves and place in a 160°C pre-heated oven for one hour.

Remove from oven, add celery, leeks, carrots and potatoes and return to oven for a further hour.

Now for the pastry – don't freak out, this is the easiest and tastiest pastry in the world!

Weigh out flour into a large bowl. Heat the milk in a pot, add the butter and allow to melt. Once the mixture has just come to the boil, pour over the flour and mix until a ball of dough is formed. That's it, job done!

Remove stew from oven, allow the mixture to cool down, season with salt and pepper, remove bay leaves and thyme stalks and add chopped parsley.

Roll out pastry to approximately 5 mm and cut in half. Line a greased pasty dish with half the pastry, fill with stew and cover with second sheet of pastry.

Crimp the edges of the pie, wash with beaten egg yolk

and bake in 180°C pre-heated oven for 35 minutes until pastry is golden brown.

Allow to cool slightly before removing from pie dish. Enjoy.

THE GRIT DOCTOR SAYS:

Calm down, break open the pie and breathe in deeply, inhaling the deliciousness therein. Try very hard to eat slowly or risk burning the roof of your mouth as, *err*, Olly did ...

Virginia's Chicken and Spicy Bean Pie

The beauty of this pie is that it is rib-stickingly delicious, full of tasty and nutritious bits and bursting with good-quality carby energy to fuel your runs!

Serve it with mash and a green veg of your choice: cabbage or broccoli. If you're trying to shift a few pounds, have it with just veg, or a baked potato if you're carb loading during your marathon training.

Serves 2. (It probably serves 3–4 restrained people but my husband and I are greedy pigs.)

Ingredients

1 packet Jus-Rol pastry (shortcrust or puff) – it
   comes in one sheet so just cut and roll
   according to your pie dish
2 chicken breasts, diced into small pieces
1 medium-sized butternut squash, peeled and
   diced small
1 small can kidney beans
1 small can haricot beans
1 big onion, finely chopped
Garlic, chopped or squished in crusher
Tomato puree, tablespoon
A good handful of grated cheddar cheese
1–1½ pints chicken or vegetable stock –
   homemade stock is tastiest if you have it, but a
   cube is fine too
Teaspoon of oregano
Chilli powder, to taste
1 bay leaf
Salt and pepper

Method

In a non-stick saucepan, add a little olive oil and gently fry
the chicken until golden on a medium heat.

Then add the onions, garlic and butternut squash and fry
for another five minutes.

Add the stock, tomato puree, kidney beans, haricot beans, bay leaves, oregano, chilli, and season to taste.

Simmer gently and let it reduce for 30 minutes on a low heat. Once it's reached the desired consistency, add the cheddar. Stir in well. You can leave this on a low heat for 15 more minutes (or much longer on the lowest heat with the pan lid on. The slower it cooks, the better it tastes).

Spoon it into a pie dish and cover with pastry. Brush well with beaten egg and bake in the oven for 35–45 minutes at 180°C. You can always use a shape cutter or a knife to cut shapes or pictures for the top of the pie. It's dead easy and always impresses if you are cooking for someone else too.

You'll know it's ready when the pastry is golden and it is bubbling away at the edges.

THE GRIT DOCTOR SAYS:

Again, peeps, remember Vig is a pro, so worry not about the shape and picture-making if the idea makes you feel quite sick. Focus your mind on cutting a great shape on race day.

I make the filling in bulk and freeze it for another time. If you are in a rush or about to go running, defrost a portion, whack a potato in the oven, go off for a run and enjoy upon your return! (You can adapt this recipe: change the meat, add any veg, beans or pulses you like. Everything works in a pie if you have meat, veg, stock and herbs – it's always a winner.)

Vig's Pasta Simplistico

1. Pasta + butter/olive oil + parmesan + black pepper
2. Pasta + butter/olive oil + parmesan + fresh basil + squeeze of fresh lemon
3. Pasta + chorizo★ + manchego/parmesan + rocket

Boil the pasta for 8 minutes until it's **al dente**. A great trick to keep it silky is to drain off the water but rather than shaking it furiously in the colander to drain off all the liquid, just drain off most of the water and then throw it straight back in the pan so it holds just a little in it. Then add any of combinations above until the cheese has melted.

Don't worry too much about quantities, just add to taste and until you get the desired consistency.

One tip when using **parmesan** with your pasta is not to add salt until you've tasted the food first as it can be quite salty already from the parmesan.

★Chorizo can vary massively in quality so you can really tell the difference if you buy a slightly more expensive one. Cheap ones from the supermarket can be really fatty and gristly. At my deli we sell a beautiful one called Chorizo Alejandro Magno which comes in a mild or a spicy version and it is TO DIE FOR. A good deli will sell something special that will make your recipe really stand out.

I love broccoli so I sometimes add some in to boost my veg intake or have a bowl of it on the side.

Pasta – use any type, but linguine or spaghetti are my favourites. Rustichella pasta is the best, which you can find in a good deli.

A GRIT DOCTOR TIP:

For marathon training, use a larger quantity of pasta than you might otherwise do – remember that you are aiming for 55–60% of your diet to be made up of carbohydrate.

Olive oil – extra virgin is the best if you have it. (**Tip** – you know you have a good olive oil if it smells like freshly cut grass. Oils like this are so good you can just enjoy warm good crusty bread dipped in to it with a little 10p-piece-size of good quality balsamic vinegar poured into the bottom. This is great with friends when you're having drinks before supper.)

THE GRIT DOCTOR SAYS:

Given how simple and easy these pasta dishes are and how much pasta you will eat while training for a marathon, it really is worth

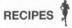
investing in some top-quality olive oil (think
how many meals one bottle will produce) and
going for the best-quality ingredients to add in.
Again, when you consider how many meals you
will get out of them, you will see how cost-
effective this kind of cooking is. If, however,
you are skint and can't tell the difference
between olive oil and castor oil anyway, don't
bother spending the extra money.

The Grit Doctor's Spaghetti *Carborama*

Pasta (al dente) + one egg yolk + splash of single cream +
parmesan + pancetta fried until crispy (or use crispy bacon
bits instead) + black pepper. Combine it all in pan until
mixed in and melted. Beware of overheating as the egg will
scramble.

I have always considered spaghetti carbonara to be a treat
food given the egg-yolky, cheesy creaminess of it and only
eat it very occasionally. I recently made it after a great friend
who has a chicken farm came to visit us armed with a dozen
double-yolkers!

21

THE FINAL WORD

Running *makes you happy . . .*

Physiologically, running makes you happy because it stimulates the release of endorphins and encourages the production of serotonin, the same hormones that are released when you fall in love, gorge on chocolate or have an orgasm. This happens both during the run and for a considerable time afterwards. You will feel a sense of contentment and well-being known as a 'runner's high'.

You will also be happy because you look so much better than all your non-running contemporaries – and both you and they know it. Guard against appearing smug about this in front of anyone who you actually like.

f you take only three things from this book let it be these:

- Run

- Drink more water

- Eat less crap

YES. WE. CAN.

I am right there beside you, struggling to run. I had to start again from scratch. Maybe not in terms of my base fitness level, but mentally I had to start from the beginning. I had zero motivation. Zero strength. Divorced from the voice of The Grit Doctor, I used every excuse in the book and added a new one: TWINS. Nine months later I had to accept it was just that – another excuse – one which could just as easily be on the list in chapter 2.

*Whatever you have going on in your life that makes you think you are different from everyone else, it is **just another excuse**. Get over it. We all have the same twenty-four hours. Singletons, couples, fat dads, thin mums, deranged mothers of multiples, young girls, old monks. Put on your trainers. Be all that you can be. Run.*

APPENDIX 1:
HEALTH AND SAFETY

GENUINE INJURY

You *know* when you have a proper injury. How? Because you are in agony. If you sprain an ankle or have properly strained a muscle, you won't be able to walk on it, let alone run. Get home and immediately apply an ice pack wrapped in a tea towel to the injured area. (Frozen peas are perfect and you will, of course, have a stack in your freezer because of your new-found love of green veg.) Don't give yourself a further injury or freeze yourself to death by holding it on for too long. Then bandage the affected area firmly and elevate it (the injured part of your body should be raised above your heart) to help reduce swelling. Anything more serious than a sprain or strain, go to the doctor and, if necessary, get a referral to a physiotherapist. And for goodness' sake, follow their instructions.

Ruth

When I went for that run after having the twins and hurt my knee, I did a very stupid thing indeed. I had a pain in my knee for a few days before I went running but I told myself it was just a twinge, it was nothing, and I went anyway. I also knew that through running, the pain would probably disappear after a few minutes because all the hormones released through running are very effective at masking aches and pains. Sure enough, ten minutes into the run I didn't feel any pain. But the relief from pain is very temporary. I woke up the next morning in agony and could not run for a long time afterwards. And I have no one to blame but my own stupid self for not listening to my body. If you have pain in your knees, for goodness' sake get it sorted before running.

PREVENTION IS BETTER THAN CURE

Don't run on concrete if you can avoid it and certainly not until you have invested in proper running shoes – these two things are your best insurance policy against injury and will help you to avoid the most common running complaints. The shoes will support your feet and ankles properly and help cushion your knees from the impact of running, which is exacerbated by running on a hard surface. While wearing the correct shoes, always warm up through walking and swinging your arms for ten minutes first and try your best to stick to grass, trails and tracks as much as possible. Rest is also important, but there's no need to overdo it. Those on my programme are getting plenty of rest anyway so don't worry about it. If, however, you have become a running nut and are nailing it six days a week, you **must have a rest day** and listen to your body.

GENERAL SAFETY

- Don't get so into your run that you try and cross roads when traffic lights are red. Jog on the spot until they turn green.

- Be aware that running on a road with an iPod is potentially risky as you can't hear approaching traffic or axe-wielding psychos. If you're running through a busy area, or anywhere where you feel uncomfortable, turn the music DOWN or better still, OFF.

- If you must run on a road, please run towards the traffic not away from it.

- Avoid running in deserted areas, especially at night.

- Don't run through a ghetto or dodgy estate unless you live in one and it's the only way out.

- Ideally, stick to well-lit, populated areas while running.

- Always carry identification in case of an accident.

- I have terrible sunspots from running without appropriate sun protection – shades, hat and sunscreen. Also try to avoid running during the hottest part of the day during the summer or while on holiday (12–3 p.m.).

- You can do yourself more harm than good by wearing knee or ankle supports without medical advice. You are most likely using them as a psychological crutch (for which The Grit Doctor has no time) and may actually be causing yourself damage in the process. Get the problem sorted by going to see your GP and getting a referral to a physiotherapist, osteopath or a podiatrist if necessary and getting the injury treated. You are not able to diagnose your knee/ankle injury yourself and sadly, nor is The Grit Doctor.

- Wear orthotics (special shoe inserts) if you have very queer feet – the assistant at the running shop will advise you on this.

- Run wearing a sports bra appropriate to the high-impact activity that running is and if you are overly well-endowed, wear two.

- Make yourself visible to passing traffic if you are running in the dark by making yourself look like a lollipop lady in light-reflective clothes – a reflective strip that goes across your front and back is ideal.

APPENDIX 2:
ONLINE RESOURCES
FOR RUNNERS

THE GRIT DOCTOR SAYS:

The Grit Doctor is not a big fan of the
internet. In the time it takes for you to Google
and faff – and then Google something else
entirely unrelated to your initial search that
looks interesting – you could have been on a
good forty-minute fat-busting run. That said,
once you have caught the running bug, the
internet is a useful place to get yourself
involved in racing, joining clubs and shopping
for kit.

FOR RACING AND RUNNING CLUBS

www.runningdiary.co.uk

www.race-calendar.com

www.runnersworld.co.uk

www.runnersweb.co.uk

www.british-athletics.co.uk/clubs

www.raceforlife.org

FOR ESTABLISHING YOUR RUNNING CIRCUIT

www.mapmyrun.com

www.mapometer.com

THE GRIT DOCTOR SAYS:
Providing it helps you get outside rather than
keeping you stuck indoors, the internet is an
incredibly useful runner's tool.

SHOE SHOPS AND OTHER SHOPS FOR RUNNERS

www.upandrunning.co.uk

www.sweatshop.co.uk

www.runandbecome.com

A GRIT DOCTOR FASHION TIP:

Be sure to buy your first running sports bra in a shop. Your sports bra size may be different from your usual bra size and the shape and feel is certainly different. It really will pay to try a few on (like the shoes) before you make up your mind. You will (perhaps) be relieved to hear that in this case, the assistant will *not* expect you to run up and down outside the shop to ensure you have the right one. Once you have got the knack, know your size and what works best for you, save yourself the time and buy them online. The time you save in going to the shops can be spent running.

And you might like to check out my own blog at www.gritdoctor.com for updates on my running adventures and the occasional bout of Grit Doctor wisdom. Or follow me on Twitter, @gritdoctor and using the hashtag #rfbr to discuss the book. Not my idea, but one forced upon me by my editor.

APPENDIX 3:
OPTIONAL RUNNING LOG

WEEK 1

Day	Task	Notes
Monday	Read Step 1 Walk 3–4 mile route	
Tuesday	REST	
Wednesday	Read Step 2 Repeat Monday	
Thursday	Read Step 3 Repeat Monday, increase pace	
Friday	REST	
Saturday	Read Step 4 Begin as Thursday. Walk first ten minutes, jog SLOWLY for five, walk remainder	
Sunday	Repeat Saturday	

WEEK 2

Day	Task	Notes
Monday	REST	
Tuesday	Walk first ten minutes, jog SLOWLY for five, walk remainder	
Wednesday	Repeat Tuesday, but extend SLOW jog to ten minutes	
Thursday	Repeat Wednesday	
Friday	REST	
Saturday	Repeat Wednesday	
Sunday	Repeat Wednesday	

WEEK 3

Ten-minute walk to warm up, followed by fifteen minutes' incredibly slow jogging, followed by walking for the remainder of the circuit without stopping. Two rest days of your choice but not consecutive to one another. Plan out your week in advance here.

Day	Task	Notes
Monday		
Tuesday		
Wednesday		
Thursday		
Friday		
Saturday		
Sunday		

WEEK 4

Ten-minute walk to warm up, followed by twenty minutes' jogging (slow down the pace of the jog if necessary to sustain it for twenty minutes), followed by walking the remainder of the circuit without stopping. Two rest days but not consecutively. Plan out your week in advance here.

Day	Task	Notes
Monday		
Tuesday		
Wednesday		
Thursday		
Friday		
Saturday		
Sunday		

WEEK 5

Ten-minute walk to warm up followed by twenty-five minutes'
jogging (slow down the pace of the jog if necessary to sustain
it for twenty minutes) followed by walking the remainder of
the circuit without stopping. Two rest days but not consecutively. Plan out your week in advance here.

Day	Task	Notes
Monday		
Tuesday		
Wednesday		
Thursday		
Friday		
Saturday		
Sunday		

WEEK 6

Ten-minute walk to warm up, followed by thirty minutes' VERY SLOW jogging, followed by walking the remainder of the circuit without stopping. Two rest days but not consecutively. Plan out your week in advance here.

Day	Task	Notes
Monday		
Tuesday		
Wednesday		
Thursday		
Friday		
Saturday		
Sunday		

WEEK 7

Ten-minute walk to warm up, followed by thirty-five minutes'
VERY SLOW jogging, followed by walking what remains of
the circuit without stopping. Two rest days but not consecutively. Plan out your week in advance here.

Day	Task	Notes
Monday		
Tuesday		
Wednesday		
Thursday		
Friday		
Saturday		
Sunday		

WEEK 8

Ten-minute walk to warm up, followed by forty minutes' VERY SLOW jogging, followed by walking home if there is anything left of the circuit. If not, always warm down by walking a few hundred metres before you go back indoors. Two rest days but not consecutively. Read and observe Step 5. Plan out your week in advance here.

Day	Task	Notes
Monday		
Tuesday		
Wednesday		
Thursday		
Friday		
Saturday		
Sunday		

APPENDIX 4:
THE GRIT DOCTOR'S ULTIMATE RUNNING PLAYLIST

The Grit Doctor prefers to run in zen-like silence, but if you need thumping basslines or cheesy 80s power ballads to get you going (like Olly), try making your own running playlist and use it to spur you on. Here are some suggestions:

For those who prefer a very literal running soundtrack

Run the World (Girls)	Beyoncé
Born to Run	Bruce Springsteen
Young Hearts Run Free	Candi Staton
Band on the Run	Wings
Running up that Hill	Kate Bush
Run to You	Bryan Adams
Run this Town	Jay-Z featuring Kanye West and Rihanna

Shoot the Runner	Kasabian
Run to the Hills	Iron Maiden
100 Miles and Running	NWA
I'm Gonna Be (500 Miles)	The Proclaimers
Run	Snow Patrol
Running to Stand Still	U2

And of course . . .

Chariots of Fire	Vangelis
Eye of the Tiger	Survivor

In a survey of fellow runners, an eclectic mix of choons came to light, ranging from hip (ish) to deeply uncool (some of which are GD faves for cutting shapes on the dancefloor★). In no particular order:

Bonkers	Dizzee Rascal *('For the adrenalin rush.')*
Rolling in the Deep	Adele
Dog Days	Florence and the Machine
Sex on Fire★	Kings of Leon *('I understand this is also the technical name for the symptoms runners can experience if they wear the wrong kind of shorts.')*

I Need a Dollar	Aloe Blacc
Common People★	Pulp
More than a Feeling	Boston
I Need a Hero	Bonnie Tyler
Don't Stop Believin'	Journey *('But it was ruined for me by* Glee . . .*')*
We Built this City	Starship
Love Shack	The B52s
Together in Electric Dreams★	Phil Oakey and Giorgio Moroder
Little Lovin'	Lissie *('For the lyric "why you runnin'?" which always makes me smile when the burn kicks in.')*
Apache	Incredible Bongo Band
I Was Drunk	Riva Starr *('Very motivating . . . somehow.')*
Time to Pretend	MGMT
Make Me Smile (Come Up and See Me)★	Steve Harley and Cockney Rebel

APPENDIX 5:
APPLYING FOR A MARATHON

The London Marathon

There are approximately 36,000 places available in the London Marathon every year and hundreds of thousands of people apply – **securing a place is not easy**. There are various ways you can apply and lots of useful information on the website. I've summarised the main information here to give you a head start.

Ballot

You can apply for a place in the London Marathon through an online ballot system:

http://www.virginlondonmarathon.com/marathon-centre/enter-virgin-london-marathon/

The ballot usually opens in April, just after that year's race. The ballot is closed once 120,000 people have applied – this usually takes no more than one day so you have to be quick. Those who are successful will find out if they have a place in October.

There are approximately 20,000 ballot places available – the remainder of the places belong to charities and athletics clubs.

Charity places

There are around 16,000 charity places available but these are also in high demand and often balloted as well. The bigger charities will have more places available but, as mentioned earlier, may be more in demand and so they may ask you to raise a higher sum of money. You have to apply directly to the charity rather than via the marathon itself, so make sure to check out the information available on the charity's website. Remember, they will ask for a reason why you want to run with them, so 'cos I want to run the marathon' isn't necessarily going to cut it – though you can apply to as many as you want.

There is a full list of charities here:

http://www.realbuzz.com/activity-listings/virgin-london-marathon/

Any other ways?

There are a couple of other ways to secure a place.

For overseas entries there are some companies who will enter you and sort out your travel:

http://london-marathon.s3.amazonaws.com/lm/pdfs/ 2013_tour_operators.pdf

If you happen to have already run a marathon in a good time (though you will need proof!), then you could automatically get in with a 'Good for Age' place. You can check the criteria here:

http://www.virginlondonmarathon.com/marathon-centre/ enter-virgin-london-marathon/good-for-age-entries/

Also, most athletics clubs have a certain number of places available, but of course you must be a member of the club and competing regularly for them at a high level.

http://www.virginlondonmarathon.com/marathon-centre/ enter-virgin-london-marathon/uk-athletics-club-entries/

Other UK marathons

It's a mistake to get hung up on London as the only marathon worth running. Of course, it's an amazing experience but it is – as we have established – quite difficult to get into and there are plenty of other brilliant marathon events all over the UK.

For a full list of UK marathons, check out this website:

http://www.marathons.org.uk/marathon-calendar/full-marathons.html

Half-marathons

Most of the full marathons listed above will also host half-marathons – often on the same course – but these are two great bespoke 13-milers.

The Great North Run

http://www.greatrun.org/events/event.aspx?id=1

Run to the Beat

http://www.runtothebeat.co.uk/

Marathons in Ireland

Clonakilty Waterfront Marathon

http://www.runclon.ie/

Connemara Marathon

http://www.connemarathon.com

Cork City Marathon

http://www.corkcitymarathon.ie/

Dingle Marathon

http://www.dinglemarathon.ie

Dublin Marathon

http://dublinmarathon.ie/

Great Limerick Run

http://www.greatlimerickrun.com/

Marathons in Australia and New Zealand

Adelaide Marathon

http://www.adelaidemarathon.com.au

Auckland Marathon, NZ

http://www.aucklandmarathon.co.nz/

Gold Coast Marathon

http://www.goldcoastmarathon.com.au/

Melbourne Marathon

http://www.melbournemarathon.com.au/

Perth Marathon

http://www.perthmarathon.com.au

Sydney Marathon

http://www.sydneyrunningfestival.com.au/

Wellington Marathon, NZ

http://www.harbourcapital.org.nz/

ACKNOWLEDGEMENTS

In no particular order: My husband, Olly, for his brilliant ideas (arguably, the title) and for humouring me. Our sons, Sebastian and Rufus (not sure for what yet). For early encouragement: Joan Johnson (1917–2010), Sacha Bonsor, Alice Lutyens, Adam Morane-Griffiths, Veronique Jackson, Louise and Roger Lamberth. All the contributors: Charlotte Pilain, Laetitia Maklouf, Jane Davies, Alice Crawford, Nicola Fister (you know who you are), Barney and Louise Oswald, Father Henry Wansbrough OSB, Chris Spira and Polly Whitton. My family: Mum, Dad, Auntie Bernadette, Pippa and Roger (for unending support and help with the twins so I could write), Simon, Peter (for the word 'grit'), Guu, Matthew and Jex. Alice Saunders (my masterful agent), Hannah Boursnell (my genius editor) and Rhiannon Smith (my extraordinary social media guru) – who I like to refer to collectively as 'my people' (as often as I can) – and everyone else at Little comma Brown. Merialeen – for looking after the twins so I could spend time with 'my people'. Sable D'Or and Caffè Nero in Muswell Hill for allowing me to make one skinny cappuccino (and the odd pain au raisin) last a whole day while writing.

If you've been inspired by The Grit Doctor,
why not try her next book:

GET YOUR SH!T TOGETHER:
Your Prescription for a Simpler Life

WHAT'S IN YOUR HANDBAG?
* To Do lists scrawled on the back of receipts
* An unpaid bill
* Half a chocolate bar, covered in fluff

Is your handbag a metaphor for the rest of your life?

Has becoming a capable, poised grown-up turned out to be
more complicated than you imagined? If you answered 'yes' to
any of these questions, and if you're tired of the crappy stuff in
life grinding you down, then it's time to stop whining and **GET
YOUR SH!T TOGETHER**. With this funny, frank and tough-
talking guide, Ruth Field and The Grit Doctor will help you:

* Tackle daunting problems like a fearless superwoman
* Figure out what you want from life and find the courage to
GO FOR IT
* Learn how to get more sh!t done in less time
* Stop feeling bad about your less-than-perfect life.
(Because perfection's overrated anyway.)

SHE TAUGHT YOU HOW TO RUN, NOW SHE'S
GOING TO TEACH YOU HOW TO RUN YOUR LIFE.

Twitter: @gritdoctor
www.gritdoctor.com